NON-PROTEINOGENIC AMINO ACIDS

Edited by **Nina Filip** and **Cristina Elena Iancu**

Non-Proteinogenic Amino Acids
http://dx.doi.org/10.5772/intechopen.71648
Edited by Nina Filip and Cristina Elena Iancu

Contributors

Kenichiro Nakashima, Mitsuhiro Wada, Shinichi Nakamura, Viji Vijayan, Sarika Gupta, Nina Filip, Cristina-Elena Iancu, Filip Cristiana, Albu Elena, Ion Hurjui, Catalina Filip, Magda Cuciureanu, Radu Florin Popa, Ovidiu Alexa, Alexandru Filip, Demetra Socolov

Notice

Statements and opinions expressed in the chapters are these of the individual contributors and not necessarily those of the editors or publisher. No responsibility is accepted for the accuracy of information contained in the published chapters. The publisher assumes no responsibility for any damage or injury to persons or property arising out of the use of any materials, instructions, methods or ideas contained in the book.

First published in London, United Kingdom, 2018 by IntechOpen
IntechOpen is the global imprint of INTECHOPEN LIMITED, registered in England and Wales, registration number: 11086078, The Shard, 25th floor, 32 London Bridge Street
London, SE19SG – United Kingdom
Printed in Croatia

British Library Cataloguing-in-Publication Data
A catalogue record for this book is available from the British Library

Additional hard copies can be obtained from orders@intechopen.com

Non-Proteinogenic Amino Acids, Edited by Nina Filip and Cristina Elena Iancu
p. cm.
Print ISBN 978-1-78984-728-4
Online ISBN 978-1-78984-729-1

We are IntechOpen,
the world's leading publisher of
Open Access books
Built by scientists, for scientists

3,900+
Open access books available

116,000+
International authors and editors

120M+
Downloads

151
Countries delivered to

Our authors are among the

Top 1%
most cited scientists

12.2%
Contributors from top 500 universities

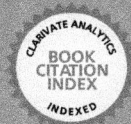

Interested in publishing with us?
Contact book.department@intechopen.com

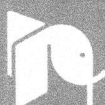

Meet the editors

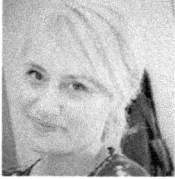

Dr. Nina Filip has been a lecturer in biochemistry, Faculty of Medicine, Grigore T. Popa University of Medicine and Pharmacy, Iaşi, since 2017. She obtained her PhD in 2010 with a thesis entitled "Biogenic amines—implications in human pathology" at the Grigore T. Popa University of Medicine and Pharmacy, Iaşi. She was a director and member of two research teams in national/international grants. Her scientific interests include the role of homocysteine in pathology, mechanisms of endothelial dysfunction in cardiovascular diseases, oxidative stress, and implications of biogenic amines in human pathology.

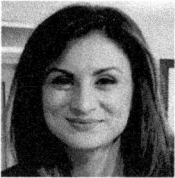

Dr. Cristina Elena Iancu has been a teaching assistant at the Department of Pharmaceutical and Clinical Biochemistry Laboratory, Grigore T. Popa University of Medicine and Pharmacy, Iaşi, since 2012. She obtained her PhD in 2016 in Pharmaceutical Sciences at the Grigore T. Popa University of Medicine and Pharmacy, Iaşi. Her scientific interests include the role of homocysteine in pathology, oxidative stress and flavonoids.

Contents

Preface

This book aims to summarize recent information on non-proteinogenic amino acids and especially homocysteine.

The chapters contain scientific works from different leading researcher groups in the field of non-proteinogenic amino acids.

The sulfur-containing amino acids and their derivatives in biological samples are quantified sensitively using high-performance liquid chromatography methods coupled with various detection methods such as UV/Vis, fluorescence, chemiluminescence, electrochemical mass spectrometry, and tandem mass spectrometry. The book includes recent advances in these analytical methods and their applications.

The book also presents information on the homocysteine metabolism and its involvement in human pathology.

In recent years, numerous studies have shown a positive correlation between serum levels and various diseases, especially vascular pathology. Vitamins B6, B12, and folic acid play a major role in controlling homocysteine levels. Homocysteine levels can be taken as an early indicator for the detection of cardiovascular diseases because Hcy levels increase after a myocardial infarction or stroke.

Over the years, numerous mechanisms have been identified through which homocysteine affects osteoblast functioning. These include alterations in collagen structure, epigenetic modifications, and changes in RANKL-OPG production by osteoblasts. These mechanisms are reviewed in this book.

This book is a significant resource for experts in basic science, biochemical pharmacologists, healthcare professionals and also other scientists who are interested in exploring the role of homocysteine in human life. We would like to express our gratitude to all the authors who had chosen to join this project by submitting their work. We would also like to thank Ms. Maja Bozicevic, Author Service Manager at InTechOpen, for her help and guidance with this work.

Nina Filip and Cristina Elena Iancu
Grigore T. Popa University of Medicine and Pharmacy
Iasi, Romania

Introduction

Chapter 1

Introductory Chapter: General Aspects Regarding Homocysteine

Nina Filip and Cristina-Elena Iancu

Additional information is available at the end of the chapter

http://dx.doi.org/10.5772/intechopen.81306

1. Historical aspect

The first description of homocysteine (Hcy), a non-proteinogenic amino acid, was introduced within a case study in 1932. The first patient was an 8-year-old child with a mental retardation disorder who died of a myocardial infarction. Meanwhile, research continued; in 1969, Dr. Kilmer McCully was the first to describe the vascular pathology in patients with homocystinuria associated with hemodynamic changes, progressive arterial stenosis, and proliferation of smooth muscle cells. He also noted that homocysteine may have a causal role in any metabolic abnormality. This idea is the basis of his theory that a moderately elevated level of homocysteine is an important risk factor for cardiovascular disease. His theory was sustained only in 1976 through a clinical trial demonstrating an increase in coronary artery disease in people with hyperhomocysteinemia. Since then, a particular interest has been given to studying this relationship.

2. Homocysteine metabolism

Homocysteine metabolism is at the crossroads of several pathways and is itself a product of the de novo pathway of the methionine metabolic reactions catalyzed by S-adenosylmethionine (SAM) and S-adenosylhomocysteine (SAH).

Homocysteine can be remethylated to methionine via the cobalamin-dependent and cobalamin-independent pathways or can be metabolized to cysteine and other metabolites via transsulfuration pathway [1]. The following enzymes are involved in the homocysteine metabolism: methionine synthase (MS), methylenetetrahydrofolate reductase (MTHFR), cystathionine β-synthase (CBS), methionine synthase reductase (MTRR), and betaine-homocysteine S-methyltransferase (BHMT).

In remethylation, homocysteine (Hcy) can be converted back to methionine in the remethylation pathway via 5-methylenetetrahydrofolate reductase (MTHFR) and methionine synthase (MS). In the transsulfuration pathway, Hcy is condensed with serine to form cystathionine via vitamin B6-dependent cystathionine β-synthase (CBS).

For proper function MS requires methylcobalamin (vitamin B12) and methionine synthase reductase (MTRR) [2]. Without MTRR, MS does not convert homocysteine into methionine.

MTHFR regulates the partitioning of folate-activated one-carbon units between the folate-dependent de novo thymidylate and homocysteine remethylation pathways. MTHFR converts 5,10-methylenetetrahydrofolate into 5-methyltetrahydrofolate (5-MTHF) required for the reaction of remethylation of homocysteine and away from thymidine synthesis. 5-Methyltetrahydrofolate acts as a substrate with vitamin B12 and S-adenosylmethionine serving as cofactors for methionine synthase. The functionality of methionine synthase is maintained by methionine synthase reductase, which catalyzes the reductive reactivation of inactive MS bound to oxidized cobalamin to maintain its active form using S-adenosylmethionine (SAM). Polymorphisms in MS and MTHFR were suggested to act independently to elevate Hcy concentrations by compromising different parts of the pathway that might not interact directly with one another [3].

The genetic variations of MTHFR have been reported to be associated with the gene deficiency and associated with susceptibility to occlusive vascular disease, neural tube defects, Alzheimer's disease, and other forms of dementia [4, 5]. In a study, C677T polymorphism in MTHFR was shown to associate with higher plasma homocysteine and the risk of brain atrophy and brain volume deficit [6]. The mutation of MTHFR results in reduced enzymatic activity and consequently accumulation of homocysteine. Plasma concentrations of folate, B12, and 5-MTHF were reduced in elderly (over 65 years old) patients with dementia [7]. There was no difference found in DNA methylation between demented patients and age-corresponding controls. However, changes in DNA methylation correlated with the folate status. Two single nucleotide polymorphisms (C677T and A1298C) in the methylenetetrahydrofolate (MTHFR) gene are important genetic predictors of Hcy level [8].

It was reported that deficit of B12, B6, and folate can lead to cognitive deficit. High level of homocysteine was observed in B12 deficiency even when the level of folate was sufficient. Only concurrent supplementation of B vitamins and folic acid has been efficient in diminishing the level of Hcy [9].

Methionine is first converted to S-adenosylmethionine, which can lose its methyl group to form S-adenosylhomocysteine (adoHcy). This demethylated product is hydrolyzed to free homocysteine which undergoes a reaction with serine, catalyzed by cystathionine β-synthase, to yield cystathionine. CBS catalyzes the pyridoxal phosphate-dependent conversion of homocysteine to cystathionine. In the animal model, it was shown that during aging the expression of CBS was not changed, whereas activity significantly decreased [10]. Subsequently, the decline in CBS activity due to nitration was attributed to observed elevated level of Hcy. High Hcy levels results from diet with an excess of methionine. In mice models it was shown that high methionine diet brings up the level of homocysteine in Cbs (+/+) and Cbs (+/−) [11].

3. Hyperhomocysteinemia and diseases

The following forms of homocysteine can be found in the plasma:

1. Free Hcy

2. Protein-bound Hcy (S-linked and N-linked)

3. Oxidized forms of Hcy   .

4. Hcy-thiolactone [1]

Hyperhomocysteinemia (HHcy) may arise from genetic defects of enzymes involved in homocysteine metabolism. There are numerous factors that influence Hcy level like age, gender, cigarette smoking, coffee and alcohol intake, and polymorphisms in genes encoding enzymes acting in one-carbon metabolism.

Hyperhomocysteinemia is defined when plasma level is more than 15 μmol/L [1]. Total concentration of homocysteine in plasma of healthy humans is low, and its level is between 5.0 and 15.0 μmol/L. Several types of HHcy are classified in relation to the total Hcy concentration: moderate (16–30 μM), intermediate (31–100 μM), and severe (higher than 100 μM) [12].

Hcy level associates with all-cause mortality risk in a linear fashion, and the risk of mortality increases for each 5 μmol/L Hcy by 33.6% [13]. In patients with heart failure, the level of Hcy reached 17.8 ± 0.7 μmol/L; Hcy reached the highest level of 20.2 ± 1.5 μmol/L in patients with cognitive impairment. Hcy exerts multiple neurotoxic mechanisms that are relevant in the development of neurodegenerative diseases such as Alzheimer's disease [14]. Hcy at the concentration over 30 μM associates with cognitive dysfunction [15]. The prevalence of hyperhomocysteinemia was significant in patients with hypertension and ischemic heart disease. Chronic hyperhomocysteinemia causes vascular remodeling by instigating vein phenotype in the artery, thus leading to cerebrovascular and vascular dysfunctions. Interestingly, a large proportion of vegetarians develop hyperhomocysteinemia and serum vitamin B12 deficiency [16]. Positive association was reported between Hcy level and physical inactivity.

A high Hcy level associates with an increased reactive oxygen species (ROS) production in the elderly [17–19]. Hcy exerts neurotoxicity by suppressing activities of Na+/K+ ATPase, superoxide dismutase (SOD), and glutathione peroxidase (GPx) and diminishing glutathione content. Redox balance disruptions and excessively generated ROS promote neuronal death in the cerebral cortex. Homocysteine (Hcy) toxicity is mediated by the posttranslational modification of proteins by its metabolite, homocysteine thiolactone (HTL). It was shown that HTL-modified cytochrome c causes conversion of the hexa-coordinate cytochrome c to a penta-coordinate species and conformational alterations affecting the packing of the apolar groups. Such changes lead to the reduction of the heme moiety and activation of peroxidase-like function of cytochrome c [20].

Clinically the measurement of homocysteine is considered important to diagnose homocystinuria to identify individuals with the risk of developing cobalamin or folate deficiency states and to assess the risk factor for young cardiovascular disease (CVD) patients (<4 years). In known cases of CVD, high homocysteine levels should be used as a prognostic marker for CVD events and mortality. Increased homocysteine levels with low vitamin concentrations should be handled as potential vitamin deficiency state. Supplementation of diets with folic acid, cobalamin, and pyridoxine appears to provide protection by lowering homocysteine levels in the blood.

The homocysteine level increases with an increasing age and is generally higher in males as compared to females. Homocysteine has been suggested to be a risk factor for fracture, but the causal relationship is not yet clear [21]. Homocysteine levels can be taken as an early indicator for the detection of cardiovascular diseases as the Hcy level increases after a myocardial infarction or stroke. No clear cut data is available that rules out homocysteine as a marker for heart disease.

Author details

Nina Filip* and Cristina-Elena Iancu

*Address all correspondence to: zamosteanu_nina@yahoo.com

Department of Biochemistry, University of Medicine and Pharmacy "Grigore T. Popa", Iasi, Romania

References

[1] Škovierová H, Vidomanová E, Mahmood S, Sopková J, Drgová A, Červeňová T, et al. The molecular and cellular effect of homocysteine metabolism imbalance on human health. International Journal of Molecular Sciences. 2016;**17**(10):1733

[2] Gaughan DJ et al. The methionine synthase reductase (MTRR) A66G polymorphism is a novel genetic determinant of plasma homocysteine concentrations. Atherosclerosis. 2001;**157**(2):451-456

[3] Ho V, Massey TE, King WD. Effects of methionine synthase and methylenetetrahydrofolate reductase gene polymorphisms on markers of one-carbon metabolism. Genes & Nutrition. 2013;**8**:571-580

[4] Efrati E, Zuckerman T, Ben-Ami E, Krivoy N. MTHFR C677T/A1298C genotype: A possible risk factor for liver sinusoidal obstruction syndrome. Bone Marrow Transplantation. 2014;**49**:726-727

[5] Mansouri L, Fekih-Mrissa N, Klai S, Mansour M, Gritli N, Mrissa R. Association of methylenetetrahydrofolate reductase polymorphisms with susceptibility to Alzheimer's disease. Clinical Neurology and Neurosurgery. 2013;**115**:1693-1696

[6] Rajagopalan P, Jahanshad N, Stein JL, Hua X, Madsen SK, et al. Common folate gene variant, MTHFR C677T, is associated with brain structure in two independent cohorts of people with mild cognitive impairment. NeuroImage: Clinical. 2012;1:179-187

[7] Bednarska-Makaruk M, Graban A, Sobczynska-Malefora A, Harrington DJ, Mitchell M, et al. Homocysteine metabolism and the associations of global DNA methylation with selected gene polymorphisms and nutritional factors in patients with dementia. Experimental Gerontology. 2016;81:83-91

[8] Misiak B, Frydecka D, Slezak R, Piotrowski P, Kiejna A. Elevated homocysteine level in first-episode schizophrenia patients—The relevance of family history of schizophrenia and lifetime diagnosis of cannabis abuse. Metabolic Brain Disease. 2014;29(3):661-670

[9] Vogel T, Dali-Youcef N, Kaltenbach G, Andres E. Homocysteine, vitamin B12, folate and cognitive functions: A systematic and critical review of the literature. International Journal of Clinical Practice. 2009;63:1061-1067

[10] Wang H, Sun Q, Zhou Y, Zhang H, Luo C, et al. Nitration-mediated deficiency of cystathionine beta-synthase activity accelerates the progression of hyperhomocysteinemia. Free Radical Biology & Medicine. 2017;113:519-529

[11] Dayal S, Bottiglieri T, Arning E, Maeda N, Malinow MR, et al. Endothelial dysfunction and elevation of S-adenosylhomocysteine in cystathionine beta-synthase-deficient mice. Circulation Research. 2001;88:1203-1209

[12] Ji C, Kaplowitz N. Hyperhomocysteinemia, endoplasmic reticulum stress, and alcoholic liver injury. World Journal of Gastroenterology. 2004;10(12):1699

[13] Fan R, Zhang A, Zhong F. Association between homocysteine levels and all-cause mortality: A dose-response meta-analysis of prospective studies. Scientific Reports. 2017;7:4769

[14] Van Dam F, Van Gool WA. Hyperhomocysteinemia and Alzheimer's disease: A systematic review. Archives of Gerontology and Geriatrics. 2009;48:425-430

[15] Bonetti F, Brombo G, Zuliani G. The relationship between hyperhomocysteinemia and neurodegeneration. Neurodegenerative Disease Management. 2016;6:133-145

[16] Obersby D, Chappell DC, Dunnett A, Tsiami AA. Plasma total homocysteine status of vegetarians compared with omnivores: A systematic review and meta-analysis. The British Journal of Nutrition. 2013;109:785-794

[17] Albu EL, Lupascu D, Filip C, Jaba IM, Zamosteanu N. The influence of a new rutin derivative on homocysteine, cholesterol and total antioxidative status in experimental diabetes in rat. Farmácia. 2013;61(6):1167-1177

[18] Filip C, Albu E, Lupascu D, Filip N. The influence of a new rutin derivative in an experimental model of induced hyperhomocysteinemia in rats. Farmácia. 2017;65(4):596-599

[19] Albu E, Filip C, Zamosteanu N, Jaba IM, Strenja-Linić I, Šoša I. Hyperhomocysteinemia is an indicator of oxidant stress. Medical Hypotheses. 2012;78(4):554-555

[20] Sharma GS, Singh LR. Conformational status of cytochrome c upon N-homocysteiny-lation: Implications to cytochrome c release. Archives of Biochemistry and Biophysics. 2017;**614**:23-27

[21] Filip A, Filip N, Veliceasa B, Filip C, Alexa O. The relationship between homocysteine and fragility fractures—A systematic review. Annual Research & Review in Biology. 2017;**16**(5):1-8

Methods for Homocysteine Analysis

Chapter 2

HPLC Analysis of Homocysteine and Related Compounds

Mitsuhiro Wada, Shinichi Nakamura and
Kenichiro Nakashima

Additional information is available at the end of the chapter

http://dx.doi.org/10.5772/intechopen.75030

Abstract

Homocysteine (Hcy), a sulfur-containing amino acid, is a representative intermediate metabolite of methionine (Met) to cysteine (Cys) via several intermediates. An elevated level of Hcy in plasma plays an important role in diseases such as neural tube defects and Down syndrome. Homocystinuria is the most common inborn error of sulfur metabolism and is caused by mutations in the metabolic enzymes of Hcy. These errors can be caused by abnormal levels of Met metabolites and classified on the basis of plasma Met levels. Additionally, Hcy and related compounds such as glutathione play an important role in maintaining homeostasis. Therefore, the simultaneous determination of Hcy and/or related compounds is required for appropriate clinical management of several diseases. The sulfur-containing amino acids and their derivatives in biological samples are quantified sensitively using high-performance liquid chromatography methods coupled with various detection methods such as UV/Vis, fluorescence, chemiluminescence, electrochemical, mass spectrometry, and tandem mass spectrometry. In this chapter, we review recent advances in these analytical methods and their applications.

Keywords: homocysteine, homocysteine-related compounds, sulfur-containing amino acids, HPLC, determination, derivatization

1. Introduction

Homocysteine (Hcy), one of the sulfur-containing amino acids, is a representative intermediate metabolite of methionine (Met) in the cysteine (Cys) biosynthetic pathway, as shown in **Figure 1**. Hcy is remethylated to Met by Met synthase or betaine-Hcy methyltransferase (transmethylation), and Met is transmethylated to Hcy via several steps. The first step in the transmethylation

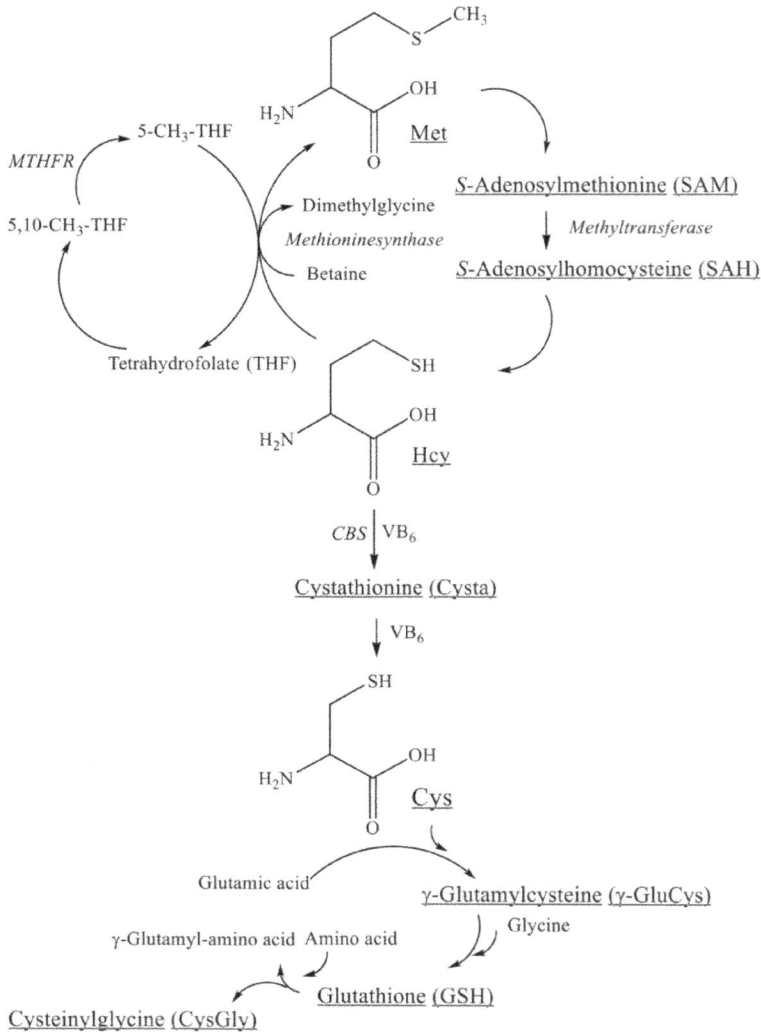

Figure 1. Relationship of Hcy and its related compounds in Met metabolism. The compounds underlined are target compounds in the references.

of Met to Hcy is the activation of Met to S-adenosylmethionine (SAM) by Met adenosyltransferase. SAM is converted to S-adenosylhomocysteine (SAH); then, SAH is hydrolyzed to Hcy by SAH hydrolase. Hcy is converted to cystathionine (Cysta) by cystathionine β-synthase (CBS) (transsulfuration); then, Cysta is hydrolyzed to Cys by cystathionine-γ-liase [1]. Cys is a fundamental substrate for glutathione (GSH) biosynthesis. In the first step of this biosynthesis, Cys and glutamate generate the dipeptide γ-glutamylcysteine (GluCys). This step is believed to be rate limiting, and enzyme activity is regulated by feedback inhibition with GSH. Next, the addition of glycine to GluCys results in the formation of GSH, catalyzed by glutathione synthase, and finally, the degradation of GSH generates cysteinylglycine (CysGly) [2, 3].

Most Hcy in human plasma is present as the bound form of Hcy, in which Hcy binds with plasma proteins through an —S—S— bond, while free Hcy is present in the oxidized or reduced form. Oxidized forms of Hcy include homocysteine (HcyHcy) and Hcy-Cys disulfide. The bound form of Hcy and the oxidized form are called S-linked Hcy. The bound form of Hcy constitutes 70–90% of the total Hcy (~10–15 μmol/L) in the body, 10–30% is present as oxidized Hcy, and less than 1% is present as reduced Hcy [4]. The ratio of Cys to Hcy in human plasma may be similar.

Hcy is metabolized to Hcy-thiolactone by methionyl-*t*RNA synthetase in an error-editing reaction during protein biosynthesis when Hcy is mistakenly replaced with Met. An increase in the Hcy level leads to elevated thiolactone levels in human cells and serum. Hcy-thiolactone reacts with proteins by N-linking to the ε-amino group of protein lysine residues (homocysteinylation), resulting in protein damage [5]. The measurement of Nε-Hcy-Lys generated by the proteolytic degradation of N-Hcy-protein provides an indicator of homocysteinylation [6].

Hcy is important for the clinical diagnosis of a variety of metabolic disorders related to human diseases. For example, an elevated Hcy plasma concentration is believed to be related to cardiovascular disease [7]. Consequently, the determination of Hcy in plasma has been used to diagnose this disease and to evaluate new diagnostic tools for atherosclerosis [8, 9]. Additionally, high plasma levels of Hcy play an important role in neural tube defects [10] and Down syndrome [11]. Homocystinuria is the most common inborn error of sulfur metabolism and is caused by homozygous mutations in the methylenetetrahydrofolate reductase (MTHFR) gene and heterozygous mutations in CBS [12]. These errors can be classified on the basis of plasma Met levels, which tend to be elevated in the case of CBS deficiency and lowered in the case of MTHFR deficiency.

DNA methylation is regulated by the Met cycle using SAM as a methyl group donor in the presence of methyltransferase. Under normal physiological conditions, SAM is hydrolyzed to adenosine and Hcy by SAH hydrolase. However, this reaction is readily reversible due to equilibrium dynamics that strongly favors SAH synthesis over hydrolysis. SAM and SAH therefore regulate the normal level of methylation in DNA, and deregulation of the methionine cycle has serious cellular consequences, resulting in disease. The ratio of SAM/SAH, called the "methylation index," may be a useful indicator of the methylation capacity of the cell [13].

Hcy toxicity appears to be the auto-oxidation of Hcy, which reduces the disulfide to a free thiol, followed by metal-independent oxidation of the free thiol to generate reactive oxygen species such as superoxide and hydrogen peroxide [14]. Therewith, other thiol compounds like Cys having a chemical structure similar to Hcy are also recognized to be risk factors of cardiovascular disease [15, 16]. In contrast, GSH is a major antioxidant and detoxifier and has many essential metabolic functions in human. GSH exists in both reduced and oxidized (GSSG) forms. CysGly is a prooxidant that reduces ferric iron to ferrous iron [17]. N-Acetylcysteine (NAC) is an endogenous product of Cys metabolism [18], and cysteamine (CA) augments intracellular Cys levels via a disulfide interchange reaction in which CA converts Cys to CA-Cys to generate Cys [19]. Homocysteine is involved in current topics, and the determination methods are useful for the researchers.

High-performance liquid chromatography (HPLC) is the most commonly used chromatographic technique for quantifying Hcy and related compounds. In contrast to gas chromatography, HPLC enables the analysis of polar and thermally labile compounds. Furthermore, HPLC can be coupled with a variety of detection methods, including ultraviolet/visible (UV/Vis), fluorescence (FL), chemiluminescence (CL), mass (or tandem mass/mass) spectrometry (MS or MS/MS), and electrochemical detection (ECD). The researcher selects the most suitable detection tools according to the aims of the analysis [20].

Several eminent reviews have been published over the past decade regarding these detection tools, e.g., HPLC-UV/Vis detection [21], HPLC-FL detection [22], HPLC-luminescence detection [23], HPLC and/or capillary electrophoresis [2, 3], electrochemical assays [24], and chromatographic methods in the study of autism [20], together with their application to the quantification of Hcy and/or related compounds and descriptions of the importance of measuring these compounds. In this chapter, we review HPLC methods and their applications in recent publications (from 2008 to 2017).

2. HPLC analysis of homocysteine and related compounds

As described above, Hcy and related compounds are found in the form of free thiols, disulfides, and protein-bound complexes and participate in metabolism, antioxidant defense, and drug detoxification. Alterations in the concentrations and ratios of free thiols and disulfides provide biomarkers of metabolism and of the redox status in biochemical, physiological, pharmacological, and toxicological studies. Therefore, analytical methods for the determination of Hcy and/or these other compounds in biological samples are extremely important. In this section we describe HPLC methods combined with various detection methods.

Pretreatment of the sample is often required for successful chromatographic analysis of Hcy and related compounds. Biological fluids such as blood (plasma or serum) and urine must be processed prior to HPLC analysis in order to (1) liberate Hcy (including the reduced disulfide), (2) provide desirable characteristics for detection, and (3) remove any interfering compounds. Sample pretreatment consists of reduction, derivatization, and/or cleanup steps. (1) The total Hcy concentration in a biological sample is important in clinical practice. Hcy can be in the reduced and in S-linked forms, such as a disulfide and Hcy bound with plasma proteins. These S-linked forms are converted to the reduced form and analyzed as the total Hcy. The disulfide can be reduced using sodium borohydride [25, 26], tributylphosphine (TBP) [27, 28], tris(2-carboxyethyl)phosphine (TCEP) [6, 29–40], dithiothreitol (DTT) [41–44], 1,4-dithioerythritol (DTE) [45–47], and mercaptoethanol [48]. Bai et al. developed a unique online reduction quartz column packed with a Zn(II)-TCEP complex [33, 49]. The column efficiently converted disulfides (except GSSH) to the reduced form as effectively as a TCEP solution. N-linked Hcy can be liberated from protein and converted to Hcy-thiolactone using harsh conditions (6 mol/L HCl at 120°C for 1 h) after removing Hcy and S-linked Hcy by reduction with DTT [36, 44]. (2) The structures of Hcy and related compounds have low absorbance and are non-fluorescent. Derivatization is therefore essential for the UV/Vis and fluorescence detection of small amounts of these compounds in biological samples. Many derivatization reagents have been developed and applied to various biological samples. Furthermore, derivatization reagents have been recently developed allowing sensitive MS or MS/MS detection for Hcy and related compounds, as described in detail below. (3) Following their reduction, Hcy and related compounds are deproteinized, then derivatized, and chromatographically separated. Cleanup is achieved using ultrafiltration [31], acid precipitation with trichloroacetic acid [28, 37, 41, 50] or perchloric acid [29, 34, 45], and organic solvent precipitation with methanol [48, 51, 52] or acetonitrile [31, 53]. Further cleanup following the derivatization of Hcy and related compounds may be required, such as a liquid-liquid extraction [45] or a solid-phase extraction [54].

2.1. UV/Vis detection

HPLC-UV/Vis is the most commonly used detection method due to the simple and relatively inexpensive instrumentation required. However, Hcy and related compounds have low absorbance and are present in biological samples in low amounts, which precludes their direct analysis by HPLC-UV/Vis. As mentioned above, this is addressed by derivatization using reagents such as those shown in **Figure 2**. The halopyridine-type derivatization reagents 2-chloro-1-methylquinolium tetrafluoroborate (CMQT) [27, 39, 40], 2-chloro-1-methyllepidinium tetrafluoroborate (CMLT) [6, 30], and 1-benzyl-2-chloropyridinium bromide (BCPB) [26] react with Hcy and related compounds to form stable S-quinolinium or S-pyridinium derivatives with intense UV

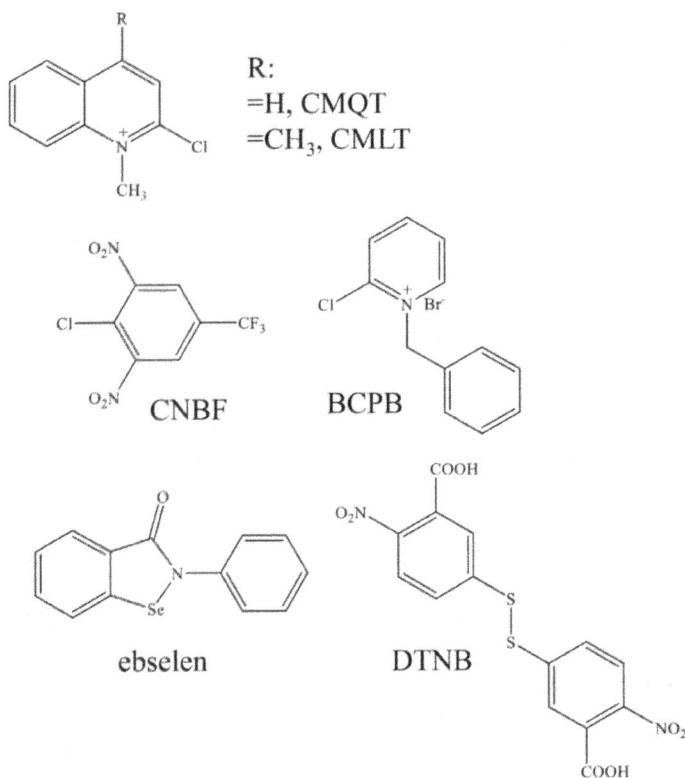

Figure 2. Chemical structures of derivatizing reagents for UV/Vis detection.

absorption. Stachniuk et al. developed an HPLC-UV/Vis method using CMLT derivatization for the determination of Hcy, Cys, GSH, GluCys, CysGly, and NAC in human saliva, plasma, and urine [30]. The analytes were separated within 7 min and monitored by absorbance at 355 nm. The limits of detection (LODs) at a signal-to-noise (S/N) ratio of 3 ranged from 0.05 to 0.12 µmol/L. The authors showed a good positive correlation between the concentrations of the analytes in plasma and saliva and suggested that saliva is an alternative to plasma for the quantification of Hcy and related compounds.

Several unique types of derivatization reagents have been reported. 4-Chloro-3,5-dinitrobenzo-trifluoride (CNBF) has an activated halide leaving group that can be easily replaced by a thiol group, leading to the formation of a stable thioether with increased absorbance at 230 nm [32]. Using this approach allowed the quantification of Hcy, Cys, CysGly, and GSH in human plasma, urine, and saliva, with LODs of 0.04–0.08 µmol/L. 5,5'-Dithiobis-2-nitrobenzoic acid (DNTP), which utilizes the sulfhydryl-disulfide exchange reaction, has been used for quantifying Hcy, Cys, CysGly, and GSH [43, 47]. Ebselen, a Se-containing derivatization reagent that reacts with the sulfhydryl group, was used for the determination of Hcy and Cys in human serum [55]. The absorbance at 254 nm of the derivatives was monitored, and separation was complete within 11 min. The derivatives could also be determined sensitively by inductively coupled plasma mass spectrometry, with an LOD of 9.6 nmol/L.

2.2. Fluorescence detection

Derivatization allows the sensitive determination of Hcy and related compounds in biological samples by FL detection. Many appropriate derivatization reagents have been developed, and representative compounds cited in this section are shown in **Figure 3**.

Halogenobenzofurazans are often used for the determination of Hcy and related compounds, with ammonium 7-fluoro-2,1,3-benzoxadiazole-4-sulfonate (SBD-F) being most commonly used. SBD derivatives are detected by FL using 385 and 515 nm for λ_{ex} and λ_{em}, respectively. Hcy, Cys, CysGly, and GSH are isocratically separated within 6 min [28]. The use of HPLC-FL under hydrophilic interaction chromatography (HILIC) conditions allows the separation of Hcy, NAC, CA, Cys, CysGly, GSH, and GluCys within 10 min. The LODs were 0.02–3.4 nmol/L at an S/N ratio of 3 [56]. The SBD-F is the standard against which newly developed methods are compared. The HPLC-FL method with SBD-F showed a good correlation with the results obtained using a bodipy-based fluorescence sensor for the determination of Hcy, Cys, and GSH in human serum [53]. In a clinical study, Hcy levels in patients with pulmonary hypertension [57], type 2 diabetes [58], and ulcerative colitis [59] were determined by HPLC-FL with SBD-F. A validated HPLC method for the routine determination of Hcy, Cys, and CA was developed [25] and applied to several hundred plasma samples. The results were used to examine the utility of carotid intima-media thickness [9] and cardio-ankle vascular index [8] as screening tools for atherosclerosis in the Japanese population. Recently, Cevasco et al. developed ammonium 5-bromo-7-fluorobenzo-2-oxa-1,3-diazol-4-sulphonate (SBD-BF) as a reagent with improved reactivity to Hcy and related compounds [37]. The reaction of SBD-BF with these substrates at room temperature is about three times faster than with SBD-F at 60°C, and Hcy, Cys, GSH, and CysGly in plasma were determined, with LODs of 0.05–20 µmol/L. 4-Fluoro-7-aminosulfonylbenzofurazan (ABD-F), another halogenobenzofurazan, was used for the determination of Hcy, Cys, GSH, and CysGly in cell culture medium [35] and plasma, urine, saliva,

	R1:	R2:
ABD-F	SO$_2$NH$_2$	H
SBD-F	SO$_3$⁻NH$_4$⁺	H
SBD-BF	SO$_3$⁻NH$_4$⁺	Br
DBD-F	SO$_2$N(CH$_3$)$_2$	H

	R$_1$:	R$_2$:
TMMB-Br	CH$_3$	CH$_2$ − Br
TMPAB-I	CH$_3$	Ph − NHCOCH$_2$I
DMDSPAB-I	CH=CH − Ph	Ph − NHCOCH$_2$I

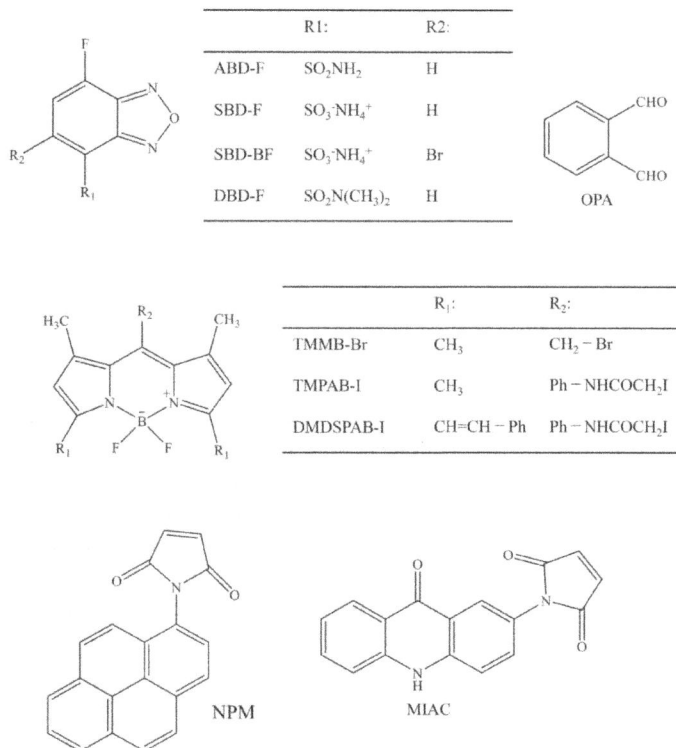

Figure 3. Chemical structures of derivatizing reagents for FL detection.

and cerebrospinal fluid [60]. The derivatization of these substrates was complete after 10 min at 35 or 50°C under alkaline conditions. FL of the ABD derivatives at around 390 and 510 nm for λ_{ex} and λ_{em} allowed sensitive determination, with LOQs of 0.1–0.5 μmol/L. Another halogeno-benzofurazan, 4-(*N,N*-dimethylaminosulfonyl)-7-fluoro-2,1,3-benzoxadiazole (DBD-F), reacts with the thiol and amino groups in Hcy and related compounds, allowing the simultaneous determination of Hcy, Cys, and Met by HPLC-FL detection and thus may be suitable for screening for homocystinuria, an inborn error of sulfur metabolism. The DBD-derivatives were separated within 15 min and quantified sensitively (0.04–0.14 μmol/L). The method was applied to maternal plasma after delivery [46] and dried blood spots from newborns [45].

o-Phthalaldehyde (OPA) is another representative derivatization reagent for Hcy and related compounds and can be used for pre- or post-column derivatization methods. Recently, Jakubowski and coresearchers developed several HPLC-FL detection methods combined with on-column derivatization for Hcy in urine [38], Hcy and Met in plasma and urine [29], and Hcy-thiolactone, *S*-linked Hcy, and *N*-linked Hcy in urine [61], plasma [36], and milk [44]. Hcy and related compounds spiked with NAC were injected and separated on a reversed-phase column, using OPA in a NaOH aqueous solution/CH$_3$CN mixture as the mobile phase. The fluorescence of the OPA-Hcy or OPA-Hcy-thiolactone derivatives generated during separation was monitored using 370 and 480 nm for λ_{ex} and λ_{em}, respectively. The LOQs for Hcy and Hcy-thiolactone were 25 [38] and 20 nmol/L [36], respectively.

Difluoroboraindacene (BODIPY) is an intense fluorogenic and stable compound, and several derivatives were recently synthesized as useful fluorescence derivatizing reagents for Hcy and related compounds. 1,3,5,7-Tetramethyl-8-bromomethyl-difluoroboradiaza-s-indacene (TMMB-Br) was used for the determination of Hcy, Cys, NAC, and GSH in human plasma [41]. The LODs ranged from 0.2 to 0.8 nmol/L by monitoring FL using 505 and 525 nm for λ_{ex} and λ_{em}. Furthermore, 1,3,5,7-tetramethyl-8-phenyl-(4-iodoacetamido)difluoroboradiaza-s-indacene (TMPAB-I) was developed for quantifying Hcy, Cys, NAC, GSH, coenzyme A [62], and 6-mercaptopurine, and 1,7-dimethyl-3,5-distyryl-8-phenyl-(4'-iodoacetamido)difluoroboradiaza-s-indacene (DMDSPAB-I) was developed for quantifying Hcy, Cys, NAC, GSH, CysGly, and penicillamine [63]. The excitation and emission wavelengths of DMDSPAB-I are very long (620 and 630 nm, respectively), which is useful for FL detection, allowing a high quantum yield of 0.557 and LODs ranging from 0.24 to 0.72 nmol/L for the substrates.

The N-substituted maleimide-type FL derivatization reagents N-(1-pyrenyl)maleimide (NPM) [31] and N-(2-acridonyl)-maleimide (MIAC) [50] were used. Among them, NPM has been applied to quantifying Hcy, Cys, CysGly, and GSH in plasma from healthy controls and uremic patients. The concentrations of the total, free, and reduced forms of Hcy, Cys, and CysGly in patients were higher than those in healthy controls, while the concentrations of the three forms of GSH were lower in the healthy controls.

A novel post-column resonance light scattering (RLS) detection method combined with HPLC was developed for quantifying Hcy and Cys in human urine [34]. Fluorosurfactant-capped gold nanoparticles (AuNPs) were used as a post-column RLS reagent. The detection principle was based on the enhanced RLS intensity of AuNPs upon the addition of Hcy or Cys (at $\lambda_{ex} = \lambda_{em} = 560$ nm).

2.3. Chemiluminescence detection

Recently, MeDermott et al. reported an HPLC-CL detection method using manganese (IV) as a post-column reagent [64]. Thiols or disulfides reacted with manganese (IV) emit red light with a maximum of 735 nm. Hcy-related compounds, including Cys, NAC, GSH, GSSG, CysCys, and HcyHcy, were determined with a single chromatographic separation. The LODs for the compounds ranged from 5×10^{-8} M to 1×10^{-7} M. This method, with simple sample pretreatment involving deproteinization, was applied to the determination of GSH and GSSG in the whole blood.

An HPLC-CL detection method using fluorosurfactant-prepared triangular gold nanoparticles (AuNPs) as a post-column CL reagent was developed for the determination of aminothiols [65]. The triangular AuNPs were generated by trisodium citrate reduction of $HAuCl_4$ in the presence of nonionic fluorosurfactant (such as zonyl FSN-100) and act as a catalyst for the luminol-H_2O_2 CL system. The reduced aminothiols decrease the CL intensity of the triangular AuNPs-luminol-H_2O_2 system. After the reduction of thiols by TCEP and deproteinization with $HClO_4$, Hcy, Cys, GSH, CysGly, and GluCys in human plasma and urine were separated by HPLC and then mixed with the AuNPs-luminol-H_2O_2 system. The LODs ranged from 0.016 to 0.1 pmol at S/N = 3. Furthermore, an automated system involving online reduction using a quartz column packed with the Zn(II)-TCEP complex was developed for quantifying

Hcy, HcyHcy, Cys, CysCys, CysGly, GSH, and GluCys [49]. The seven compounds in human plasma and urine could be determined, with LODs in the range of 8.3–25.4 nmol/L.

2.4. Electrochemical detection

ECD methods are suitable for the detection of Hcy and related compounds due to the electrochemical activity of these compounds, allowing thiols to be directly detected without derivatization. This detection method is frequently used because of the simplicity, inexpensiveness, and sensitivity of the instruments and the approach. Furthermore, the disulfide compound can be detected without cleavage of the disulfide bond.

Khan et al. reported an HPLC-ECD method for the simultaneous determination of Hcy, Met, Cys, CysCys, GSH, GSSH, NAC, and ascorbic acid (ASA) in human plasma and erythrocytes using dopamine as an internal standard (IS) [66]. The analytes were extracted from the biological fluids by simple liquid-liquid extraction. The nine compounds and the IS were separated within 25 min, and their LODs ranged from 0.6 to 25 ng/mL at an S/N ratio of 3. Furthermore, an ion-pairing reversed-phase-HPLC-ECD method was reported [67] in which total Cys, Hcy, and GSH were reduced by TCEP, and Met and ASA in human plasma and blood cell were determined with LODs of 60–80 pg/mL in a total analysis time of 20 min. More recently, Hannan et al. reported an HPLC-ECD method for nine compounds and malondialdehyde in rabbit serum [68], allowing the endogenous antioxidant capacity and lipid peroxidation level to be monitored simultaneously.

Lehotay's research group reported a two-dimensional HPLC-ECD method for determination of the enantiomers of Hcy, Cys, and Met using a combination of ODS and teicoplanin aglycone columns [69, 70]. The chiral separation of Hcy, Cys, and Met enantiomers was realized in a single 130 min analytical run. The D-enantiomers were more strongly retained by the chiral selector than the L-enantiomers, and the LODs of the method ranged from 0.05 to 0.5 µg/mL. As a clinical application, the amino acid enantiomers in the serum of healthy volunteers and multiple sclerosis patients were determined. The D-enantiomers of the amino acids were not detected in all samples, but the total L-Met levels in the patients were significantly higher than those in the healthy subjects. An improved method using a teicoplanin aglycone column separated the enantiomers using an ion-pairing reversed-phase mode and a low column temperature [71].

2.5. Mass spectrometry or tandem mass spectrometry detection

HPLC-MS and HPLC-MS/MS are characterized by high sensitivity and rapid separation which enables the efficient and accurate analysis of biological samples. Recently, several methods for the direct or indirect (with derivatization) determination of Hcy and related compounds have been developed.

2.5.1. Direct analysis

Several HPLC-ESI-MS or HPLC-MS/MS methods for determination of the total Hcy concentration in a blood sample (plasma or serum) have been developed. Hcy was reduced with suitable reagents; then sample preparation was completed with a simple deproteinization step [48, 52]. Wang et al. reported a method for the sensitive determination of compounds related to Hcy metabolism, such as Hcy, Met, SAM, SAH, Cysta, FA, THF, 5-MT, 5-FT, serine, and histidine in human serum [72], with LODs of 0.05–1 ng/mL. Using this method, 96 serum samples comprising 46 neural tube defect cases and 50 controls were analyzed. The results showed that SAH is a risk factor for neural tube defects. Another HPLC-ESI-MS/MS method for quantifying Hcy, Cys, SAM, SAH, Cysta, Met, GSH, and CysGly in plasma using N-(2-mercaptopropionyl)-glycine as an IS was used to identify biomarkers for diabetic nephropathy [51].

An HPLC-ESI-MS/MS method for the determination of SAM and SAH in cultures of ovarian cancer cells was developed [13]. LODs of approximately 0.5 ng/mL for both targeted analytes allowed the designed strategy to evaluate the effect of cisplatin on changes in the methylation index between epithelial ovarian cell lines sensitive to (A2780) and resistant to (A2780CIS) to this drug after exposure to cisplatin. In addition, a stable-isotope dilution UPLC-MS/MS method for both compounds has been reported [54]. This method showed high sensitivity (0.5 for SAM and 0.7 nmol/L for SAH) and selectivity, low RSD (less than 3.3 RSD% for intra-assays and less than 10.1 RSD% for inter-assays), fast sample preparation (40 samples in 60 min), and a short analysis run time (3 min).

Urinary Hcy sulfonic acid is a biomarker candidate for diseases used in metabolomics approaches and was quantified by HPLC coupled with time-of-flight mass spectrometric detection (-Q-TOF/MS). An increase in Hcy sulfonic acid concentration in the urine of patients with nephrolithiasis was caused by melamine [73], and a decrease was observed in pregnant patients with intrahepatic cholestasis [74] compared with healthy volunteers.

2.5.2. Derivatization methods

HPLC-MS (or HPLC-MS/MS) detection is often used for the determination of compounds in biological samples, but the sensitivity of this method can be inadequate due to low ionization efficiency of the analyzed specimen. Hcy and related compounds ionize poorly in comparison with other amino acids, and thus the introduction of nucleophilic groups and/or hydrophobic residues into these compounds might be useful. Derivatization reagents used to make the thiol group resistant to oxidation are shown in **Figure 4**. N-Ethylmaleimide (NEM) was used for the determination of Hcy in human plasma using an HPLC-MS system. The total and reduced (using DTT) concentrations of Hcy were determined with an LOD of 10 nM. Furthermore, HPLC-Orbitrap MS methods combined with p-(hydroxymercuri)benzoate (PHMB) as an organic mercury derivatization reagent were developed. The levels in yeast of Hcy, Cys, GSH, CysGLy, GluCys, and SAH, reduced using TCEP, were determined [75]. The derivatives could be detected by HPLC-ICP-MS, but the LODs (12–128 fmol/injection) and precision for the Orbitrap MS method are higher than those of the HPLC-ICP-MS method (440–1100 fmol/injection) [17]. Thirty-six amino acids, including Hcy, Met, Hcy-Cys disulfide, Cys, Met-sulfone, Met-sulfoxide, HcyHcy, and CysCys, were determined after post-column derivatization with ninhydrin [76]. The derivatized amino acids were separated on a hydrophilic interaction liquid chromatography column with an analysis time of 18 min and LODs of 0.1 µmol/L. As a clinical application, 97 plasma samples were analyzed for inborn errors of amino acid metabolism. An

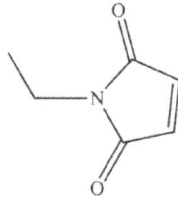

N-ethylmaleimide (NEM)

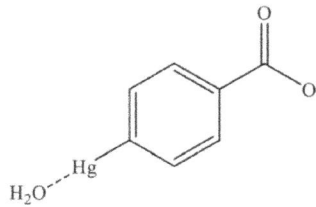

p-hydroxymercuribenzoate (PHMB)

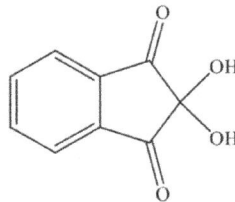

ninhydrin

Figure 4. Chemical structures of derivatizing reagents for MS or MS/MS detection.

increase or decrease in metabolites was identified in 95 of the samples, providing a clinical sensitivity of 97.9%.

3. Conclusions

HPLC methods coupled with various detection methods reported over the past decade were reviewed, focusing on their application for the determination of Hcy and related compounds. FL detection methods combined with novel or traditional derivatization reagents remain important for clinical studies. Also, UV/Vis and ECD are powerful, highly sensitive methods for analyzing biological samples. MS and MS/MS detection are powerful tools for identifying biomarkers of disease using a metabolomics approach. Further development of methods in the next decade by analytical researchers is anticipated.

Conflict of interest

The authors have declared no conflict of interest.

Author details

Mitsuhiro Wada[1]*, Shinichi Nakamura[1] and Kenichiro Nakashima[2]

*Address all correspondence to: m-wada@phoenix.ac.jp

1 School of Pharmaceutical Sciences, Kyushu University of Health and Welfare, Nobeoka, Miyazaki, Japan

2 Faculty of Pharmaceutical Sciences, Nagasaki International University, Sasebo, Nagasaki, Japan

References

[1] Perła-Kaján J, Twardowski T, Jakubowski H. Mechanisms of homocysteine toxicity in humans. Amino Acids. 2007;**32**:561-572. DOI: 10.1007/s00726-006-0432-9

[2] Kuśmierek K, Chwatko G, Głowacki R, Kubalczyk P, Bald E. Ultraviolet derivatization of low-molecular-mass thiols for high performance liquid chromatography and capillary electrophoresis analysis. Journal of Chromatography B: Analytical Technologies in the Biomedical and Life Sciences. 2011;**879**:1290-1307. DOI: 10.1016/j.jchromb.2010.10.035

[3] Isokawa M, Kanamori T, Funatsu T, Tsunoda M. Analytical methods involving separation techniques for determination of low-molecular-weight biothiols in human plasma and blood. Journal of Chromatography B: Analytical Technologies in the Biomedical and Life Sciences. 2014;**964**:103-115. DOI: 10.1016/j.jchromb.2013.12.041

[4] Refsum H, Ueland PM, Nygård O, Vollset SE. Homocysteine and cardiovascular disease. Annual Review of Medicine. 1998;**49**:31-62. DOI: 10.1146/annurev.med.49.1.31

[5] Jakubowski H. Homocysteine thiolactone: Metabolic origin and protein homocysteinylation in humans. Journal of Nutrition. 2000;**130**:377S-381S

[6] Głowacki R, Borowczyk K, Bald E. Determination of $N\varepsilon$-homocysteinyl-lysine and γ-glutamylcysteine in plasma by liquid chromatography with UV-detection. Journal of Analytical Chemistry. 2014;**69**:583-589. DOI: 10.1134/S1061934814060082

[7] Boushey CJ, Beresford SA, Omenn GS, Motulsky AG. A quantitative assessment of plasma homocysteine as a risk factor for vascular disease. Probable benefits of increasing folic acid intakes. Journal of the American Medical Association. 1995;**274**:1049-1057

[8] Kadota K, Takamura N, Aoyagi K, Yamasaki H, Usa T, Nakazato M, Maeda T, Wada M, Nakashima K, Abe K, Takeshima F, Ozono Y. Availability of cardio-ankle vascular index

(CAVI) as a screening tool for atherosclerosis. Circulation Journal. 2008;**72**:304-308. DOI: 10.1253/circj.72.304

[9]   Takamura N, Abe Y, Nakazato M, Maeda T, Wada M, Nakashima K, Kusano Y, Aoyagi K. Determinants of plasma homocysteine levels and carotid intima-media thickness in Japanese. Asian Pacific Journal of Clinical Nutrition. 2007;**16**:698-703

[10] Mills JL, Scott JM, Kirke PN, McPartlin JM, Conley MR, Weir DG, Molloy AM, Lee YJ. Homocysteine and neural tube defects. Journal of Nutrition. 1996;**126**:756S-760S

[11] Coppedè F. The complex relationship between folate/homocysteine metabolism and risk of Down syndrome. Mutation Research. 2009;**682**:54-70. DOI: 10.1016/j.mrrev.2009.06.001

[12] Melnyk S, Pogribna M, Pogribny I, Hine RJ, James SJ. A new HPLC method for the simultaneous determination of oxidized and reduced plasma aminothiols using coulometric electrochemical detection. Journal of Nutritional Biochemistry. 1999;**10**:490-497

[13] Iglesias González T, Cinti M, Montes-Bayón M, Fernández de la Campa MR, Blanco-González E. Reversed phase and cation exchange liquid chromatography with spectrophotometric and elemental/molecular mass spectrometric detection for *S*-adenosyl methionine/*S*-adenosyl homocysteine ratios as methylation index in cell cultures of ovarian cancer. Journal of Chromatography A. 2015;**1393**:89-95. DOI: 10.1016/j.chroma.2015.03.028

[14] Hogg N. The effect of cyst(e)ine on the auto-oxidation of homocysteine. Free Radical Biology and Medicine. 1999;**27**:28-33

[15] Kumar A, John L, Alam MM, Gupta A, Sharma G, Pillai B, Sengupta S. Homocysteine- and cysteine-mediated growth defect is not associated with induction of oxidative stress response genes in yeast. Biochemical Journal. 2006;**396**:61-69. DOI: 10.1042/BJ20051411

[16] Wronska-Nofer T, Nofer JR, Stetkiewicz J, Wierzbicka M, Bolinska H, Fobker M, Schulte H, Assmann G, von Eckardstein A. Evidence for oxidative stress at elevated plasma thiol levels in chronic exposure to carbon disulfide (CS2) and coronary heart disease. Nutrition, Metabolism and Cardiovascular Diseases. 2007;**17**:546-553. DOI: 10.1016/j. numecd.2006.03.002

[17] Bakirdere S, Bramanti E, D'ulivo A, Ataman OY, Mester Z. Speciation and determination of thiols in biological samples using high performance liquid chromatography-inductively coupled plasma-mass spectrometry and high performance liquid chromatography-Orbitrap MS. Analytica Chimica Acta. 2010;**680**:41-47. DOI: 10.1016/j.aca.2010.09.023

[18] Schmidt LE, Knudsen TT, Dalhoff K, Bendtsen F. Effect of acetylcysteine on prothrombin index in paracetamol poisoning without hepatocellular injury. Lancet. 2002;**360**:1151-1152. DOI: 10.1016/S0140-6736(02)11194-9

[19] Wood PL, Khan MA, Moskal JR. Cellular thiol pools are responsible for sequestration of cytotoxic reactive aldehydes: central role of free cysteine and cysteamine. Brain Research. 2007;**1158**:158-163. DOI: 10.1016/j.brainres.2007.05.007

[20] Zurawicz E, Kaluzna-Czaplińska J, Rynkowski J. Chromatographic methods in the study of autism. Biomedical Chromatography. 2013;**27**:1273-1279. DOI: 10.1002/bmc.2911

[21] Kuśmierek K, Chwatko G, Głowacki R, Bald E. Determination of endogenous thiols and thiol drugs in urine by HPLC with ultraviolet detection. Journal of Chromatography B: Analytical Technologies in the Biomedical and Life Sciences. 2009;**877**:3300-3308. DOI: 10.1016/j.jchromb.2009.03.038

[22] Guo XF, Wang H, Guo YH, Zhang ZX, Zhang HS. Simultaneous analysis of plasma thiols by high-performance liquid chromatography with fluorescence detection using a new probe, 1,3,5,7-tetramethyl-8-phenyl-(4-iodoacetamido)difluoroboradiaza-*s*-indacene. Journal of Chromatography A. 2009;**1216**:3874-3880. DOI: 10.1016/j.chroma.2009.02.083

[23] Nakashima K. Development and application of sensitive methods with luminescence detections for determination of biologically active compounds. Journal of Health Science. 2011;**57**:10-21. DOI: 10.1248/jhs.57.10

[24] Baron M, Sochor J. Estimation of thiol compounds cysteine and homocysteine in sources of protein by means of electrochemical techniques. International Journal of Electrochemical Science. 2013;**8**:11072-11086

[25] Ichinose S, Nakamura M, Maeda M, Ikeda R, Wada M, Nakazato M, Ohba Y, Takamura N, Maeda T, Aoyagi K, Nakashima K. A validated HPLC-fluorescence method with a semi-micro column for routine determination of homocysteine, cysteine and cysteamine, and the relation between the thiol derivatives in normal human plasma. Biomedical Chromatography. 2009;**23**:935-939. DOI: 10.1002/bmc.1205

[26] Kuśmierek K, Bald E. Reversed-phase liquid chromatography method for the determination of total plasma thiols after derivatization with 1-benzyl-2-chloropyridinium bromide. Biomedical Chromatography. 2009;**23**:770-775. DOI: 10.1002/bmc.1183

[27] Khalighi HR, Mortazavi H, Alipour S, Nadizadeh K. Relationship between salivary and plasma level of homocysteine in coronary artery disease. Dental and Medical Problems. 2015;**52**:22-25

[28] Ferin R, Pavão ML, Baptista J. Methodology for a rapid and simultaneous determination of total cysteine, homocysteine, cysteinylglycine and glutathione in plasma by isocratic RP-HPLC. Journal of Chromatography B: Analytical Technologies in the Biomedical and Life Sciences. 2012;**911**:15-20. DOI: 10.1016/j.jchromb.2012.10.022

[29] Borowczyk K, Chwatko G, Kubalczyk P, Jukubowski H, Kubalska J, Głowacki R. Simultaneous determination of methionine and homocysteine by on-column derivatization with *o*-phtaldialdehyde. Talanta. 2016;**161**:917-924. DOI: 10.1016/j.talanta.2016.09.039

[30] Stachniuk J, Kubalczyk P, Furmaniak P, Głowacki RA. Versatile method for analysis of saliva, plasma and urine for total thiols using HPLC with UV detection. Talanta. 2016;**155**:70-77. DOI: 10.1016/j.talanta.2016.04.031

[31] Ma L, He J, Zhang X, Cui Y, Gao J, Tang X, Ding M. Determination of total, free, and reduced homocysteine and related aminothiols in uremic patients undergoing hemodialysis by precolumn derivatization HPLC with fluorescence detection. RSC Advances. 2014;**4**:58412-58416. DOI: 10.1039/c4ra10138c

[32] Zhang W, Li P, Geng Q, Duan Y, Guo M, Cao Y. Simultaneous determination of glutathione, cysteine, homocysteine, and cysteinylglycine in biological fluids by ion-pairing high-performance liquid chromatography coupled with precolumn derivatization. Journal of Agricultural and Food Chemistry. 2014;**62**:5845-5852. DOI: 10.1021/jf5014007

[33] Zhang L, Lu B, Lu C, Lin JM. Determination of cysteine, homocysteine, cystine, and homocystine in biological fluids by HPLC using fluorosurfactant-capped gold nanoparticles as postcolumn colorimetric reagents. Journal of Separation Science. 2014;**37**:30-36. DOI: 10.1002/jssc.201300998

[34] Xiao Q, Gao H, Yuan Q, Lu C, Lin JM. High-performance liquid chromatography assay of cysteine and homocysteine using fluorosurfactant-functionalized gold nanoparticles as postcolumn resonance light scattering reagents. Journal of Chromatography A. 2013; **1274**:145-150. DOI: 10.1016/j.chroma.2012.12.016

[35] Steele ML, Ooi L, Münch G. Development of a high-performance liquid chromatography method for the simultaneous quantitation of glutathione and related thiols. Analytical Biochemistry. 2012;**429**:45-52. DOI: 10.1016/j.ab.2012.06.023

[36] Głowacki R, Bald E, Jakubowski H. An on-column derivatization method for the determination of homocysteine-thiolactone and protein N-linked homocysteine. Amino Acids. 2011;**41**:187-194. DOI: 10.1007/s00726-010-0521-7

[37] Cevasco G, Piatek AM, Scapolla C, Thea S. An improved method for simultaneous analysis of aminothiols in human plasma by high-performance liquid chromatography with fluorescence detection. Journal of Chromatography A. 2010;**1217**:2158-2162. DOI: 10.1016/j.chroma.2010.02.012

[38] Głowacki R, Borowczyk K, Bald E, Jakubowski H. On-column derivatization with o-phthaldialdehyde for fast determination of homocysteine in human urine. Analytical and Bioanalytical Chemistry. 2010;**396**:2363-2366. DOI: 10.1007/s00216-010-3456-7

[39] Gowacki R, Bald E. Determination of n-acetylcysteine and main endogenous thiols in human plasma by HPLC with ultraviolet detection in the form of their s-quinolinium derivatives. Journal of Liquid Chromatography and Related Technologies. 2009;**32**:2530-2544. DOI: 10.1080/10826070903249666

[40] Głowacki R, Bald E. Fully automated method for simultaneous determination of total cysteine, cysteinylglycine, glutathione and homocysteine in plasma by HPLC with UV absorbance detection. Journal of Chromatography B: Analytical Technologies in the Biomedical and Life Sciences. 2009;**877**:3400-3404. DOI: 10.1016/j.jchromb.2009.06.012

[41] Guo XF, Zhu H, Wang H, Zhang HS. Determination of thiol compounds by HPLC and fluorescence detection with 1,3,5,7-tetramethyl-8-bromomethyl-difluoroboradiaza-s-indacene. Journal of Separation Science. 2013;**36**:658-664. DOI: 10.1002/jssc.201200936

[42] Ivanov AV, Luzyanin BP, Kubatiev AA. The use of N-ethylmaleimide for mass spectrometric detection of homocysteine fractions in blood plasma. Bulletin of Experimental Biology and Medicine. 2012;**152**:289-292. DOI: 10.1007/s10517-012-1510-5

[43] Alkaraki AK, Hunaiti AA, Sadiq MF. Simultaneous aminothiol determination in Down syndrome individuals using a modified HPLC method. International Journal of Integrative Biology. 2010;**10**:90-93

[44] Jakubowski H. New method for the determination of protein *N*-linked homocysteine. Analytical Biochemistry. 2008;**380**:257-261. DOI: 10.1016/j.ab.2008.05.049

[45] Wada M, Kuroki M, Minami Y, Ikeda R, Sekitani Y, Takamura N, Kawakami S, Kuroda N, Nakashima K. Quantitation of sulfur-containing amino acids, homocysteine, methionine and cysteine in dried blood spot from newborn baby by HPLC-fluorescence detection. Biomedical Chromatography. 2014;**28**:810-814. DOI: 10.1002/bmc.3142

[46] Wada M, Hirose M, Kuroki M, Ikeda R, Sekitani Y, Takamura N, Kuroda N, Nakashima K. Simultaneous determination of homocysteine, methionine and cysteine in maternal plasma after delivery by HPLC-fluorescence detection with DBD-F as a label. Biomedical Chromatography. 2013;**27**:708-713. DOI: 10.1002/bmc.2848

[47] Özyürek M, Baki S, Güngör N, Çelik SE, Güçlü K, Apak R. Determination of biothiols by a novel on-line HPLC-DTNB assay with post-column detection. Analytica Chimica Acta. 2012;**750**:173-181. DOI: 10.1016/j.aca.2012.03.056

[48] Ivanov AV, Luzyanin BP, Moskovtsev AA, Rotkina AS, Kubatiev AA. Determination of total homocysteine in blood plasma by capillary electrophoresis with mass spectrometry detection. Journal of Analytical Chemistry. 2011;**66**:317-321. DOI: 10.1134/S1061934811030075

[49] Bai S, Chen Q, Lu C, Lin JM. Automated high performance liquid chromatography with on-line reduction of disulfides and chemiluminescence detection for determination of thiols and disulfides in biological fluids. Analytica Chimica Acta. 2013;**768**:96-101. DOI: 10.1016/j.aca.2013.01.035

[50] Benkova B, Lozanov V, Ivanov IP, Todorava A, Milanov I, Mitev V. Determination of plasma aminothiols by high performance liquid chromatography after precolumn derivatization with *N*-(2-acridonyl)maleimide. Journal of Chromatography B: Analytical Technologies in the Biomedical and Life Sciences. 2008;**870**:103-108. DOI: 10.1016/j.jchromb.2008.06.015

[51] Jiang Z, Liang Q, Luo G, Hu P, Li P, Wang Y. HPLC-electrospray tandem mass spectrometry for simultaneous quantitation of eight plasma aminothiols: Application to studies of diabetic nephropathy. Talanta. 2009;**77**:1279-1284. DOI: 10.1016/j.talanta.2008.08.031

[52] Persichilli S, Gervasoni J, Iavarone F, Zuppi C, Zappacosta B. A simplified method for the determination of total homocysteine in plasma by electrospray tandem mass spectrometry. Journal of Separation Science. 2010;**33**:3119-3124. DOI: 10.1002/jssc.201000399

[53] Jia M-Y, Niu L-Y, Zhang Y, Yang Q-Z, Tung C-H, Guan Y-F, Feng L. BODIPY-based fluorometric sensor for the simultaneous determination of Cys, Hcy, and GSH in human serum. ACS Applied Materials and Interfaces. 2015;**7**:5907-5914. DOI: 10.1021/acsami.5b00122

[54] Kirsch SH, Knapp JP, Geisel J, Herrmann W, Obeid R. Simultaneous quantification of S-adenosyl methionine and S-adenosyl homocysteine in human plasma by stable-isotope dilution ultra performance liquid chromatography tandem mass spectrometry. Journal of Chromatography B: Analytical Technologies in the Biomedical and Life Sciences. 2009;**877**:3865-3870. DOI: 10.1016/j.jchromb.2009.09.039

[55] Espina JG, Montes-Bayón M, Blanco-González E, Sanz-Medel A. Determination of reduced homocysteine in human serum by elemental labelling and liquid chromatography with ICP-MS and ESI-MS detection. Analytical and Bioanalytical Chemistry. 2015;**407**:7899-7906. DOI: 10.1007/s00216-015-8956-z

[56] Isokawa M, Funatsu T, Tsunoda M. Fast and simultaneous analysis of biothiols by high-performance liquid chromatography with fluorescence detection under hydrophilic interaction chromatography conditions. The Analyst. 2013;**138**:3802-3808. DOI: 10.1039/c3an00527e

[57] Costa De Campos Barbosa TM, Das Graças Carvalho M, Nicácio Silveira J, Rios JG, Komatsuzaki F, Carvalho Godói L, Yoshizane Costa GH. Homocysteine: Validation and comparison of two methods using samples from patients with pulmonary hypertension. Jornal Brasileiro de Patologia e Medicina Laboratorial. 2014;**50**:402-409. DOI: 10.5935/1676-2444.20140048

[58] Valente A, Bronze MR, Bicho M, Duarte R, Costa HS. Validation and clinical application of an UHPLC method for simultaneous analysis of total homocysteine and cysteine in human plasma. Journal of Separation Science. 2012;**35**:3427-3433. DOI: 10.1002/jssc.201200672

[59] Chen M, Mei Q, Xu J, Lu C, Fang H, Liu X. Detection of melatonin and homocysteine simultaneously in ulcerative colitis. Clinica Chimica Acta. 2012;**413**:30-33. DOI: 10.1016/j.cca.2011.06.036

[60] Persichilli S, Gervasoni J, Castagnola M, Zuppi C, Zappacosta B. A reversed-phase HPLC fluorimetric method for simultaneous determination of homocysteine-related thiols in different body fluids. Laboratory Medicine. 2011;**42**:657-662. DOI: 10.1309/LMOIAH19RG5BKBIQ

[61] Jakubowski H. Quantification of urinary S- and N-homocysteinylated protein and homocysteine-thiolactone in mice. Analytical Biochemistry. 2016;**508**:118-123. DOI: 10.1016/j.ab.2016.06.002

[62] McMenamin ME, Himmelfarb J, Nolin TD. Simultaneous analysis of multiple aminothiols in human plasma by high performance liquid chromatography with fluorescence detection. Journal of Chromatography B: Analytical Technologies in the Biomedical and Life Sciences. 2009;**877**:3274-3281. DOI: 10.1016/j.jchromb.2009.05.046

[63] Zhang L-Y, Tu F-Q, Guo X-F, Wang H, Wang P, Zhang H-S. A new BODIPY-based long-wavelength fluorescent probe for chromatographic analysis of low-molecular-weight thiols. Analytical and Bioanalytical Chemistry. 2014;**406**:6723-6733. DOI: 10.1007/s00216-014-8013-3

[64] McDermott GP, Terry JM, Conlan XA, Barnett NW, Francis PS. Direct detection of biologically significant thiols and disulfides with manganese(IV) chemiluminescence. Analytical Chemistry. 2011;**83**:6034-6039. DOI: 10.1021/ac2010668

[65] Li Q, Shang F, Lu C, Zheng Z, Lin JM. Fluorosurfactant-prepared triangular gold nanoparticles as postcolumn chemiluminescence reagents for high-performance liquid chromatography assay of low molecular weight aminothiols in biological fluids. Journal of Chromatography A. 2011;**1218**:9064-9070. DOI: 10.1016/j.chroma.2011.10.021

[66] Khan A, Khan MI, Iqbal Z, Shah Y, Ahmad L, Nazir S, Wason DG, Khan JA, Nasir F, Ismail. A new HPLC method for the simultaneous determination of ascorbic acid and aminothiols in human plasma and erythrocytes using electrochemical detection. Talanta. 2011;**84**:789-801. DOI: 10.1016/j.talanta.2011.02.019

[67] Khan MI, Iqbal Z. Simultaneous determination of ascorbic acid, aminothiols, and methionine in biological matrices using ion-pairing RP-HPLC coupled with electrochemical detector. Journal of Chromatography B: Analytical Technologies in the Biomedical and Life Sciences. 2011;**879**:2567-2575. DOI: 10.1016/j.jchromb.2011.07.013

[68] Hannan PA, Khan JA, Iqbal Z, Ullah I, Rehman UW, Rehman M, Nasir F, Khan A, Muhammad S, Hassan M. Simultaneous determination of endogenous antioxidants and malondialdehyde by RP-HPLC coupled with electrochemical detector in serum samples. Journal of Liquid Chromatography and Related Technologies. 2015;**38**:1052-1060. DOI: 10.1080/10826076.2015.1012522

[69] Deáková Z, Duráckóva Z, Armstrong DW, Lehotay J. Separation of enantiomers of selected sulfur-containing amino acids by using serially coupled achiral-chiral columns. Journal of Liquid Chromatography and Related Technologies. 2015;**38**:789-794. DOI: 10.1080/10826076.2014.968666

[70] Deáková Z, Duráckóva Z, Armstrong DW, Lehotay J. Two-dimensional high performance liquid chromatography for determination of homocysteine, methionine and cysteine enantiomers in human serum. Journal of Chromatography A. 2015;**1408**:118-124. DOI: 10.1016/j.chroma.2015.07.009

[71] Bystrická Z, Bystrický R, Lehotay J. Thermodynamic study of HPLC enantioseparations of some sulfur-containing amino acids on teicoplanin columns in ion-pairing reversed-phase mode. Journal of Liquid Chromatography and Related Technologies. 2016;**39**:775-781. DOI: 10.1080/10826076.2016.1247715

[72] Wang Y, Zhang HY, Liang QL, Yang HH, Wang YM, Liu QF, Hu P, Zheng XY, Song XM, Chen G, Zhang T, Wu JX, Luo GA. Simultaneous quantification of 11 pivotal metabolites in neural tube defects by HPLC-electrospray tandem mass spectrometry. Journal of Chromatography B: Analytical Technologies in the Biomedical and Life Sciences. 2008;**863**:94-100. DOI: 10.1016/j.jchromb.2008.01.010

[73] Duan H, Guan N, Wu Y, Zhang J, Ding J, Shao B. Identification of biomarkers for melamine-induced nephrolithiasis in young children based on ultra high performance

liquid chromatography coupled to time-of-flight mass spectrometry (U-HPLC-Q-TOF/MS). Journal of Chromatography B: Analytical Technologies in the Biomedical and Life Sciences. 2011;**879**:3544-3550. DOI: 10.1016/j.jchromb.2011.09.039

[74] Ma L, Zhang X, Pan F, Cui Y, Yang T, Deng L, Shao Y, Ding M. Urinary metabolomic analysis of intrahepatic cholestasis of pregnancy based on high performance liquid chromatography/mass spectrometry. Clinica Chimica Acta. 2017;**471**:292-297. DOI: 10.1016/j.cca.2017.06.021

[75] Rao Y, Xiang B, Bramanti E, D'Ulivo A, Mester Z. Determination of Thiols in Yeast by HPLC coupled with LTQ-Orbitrap mass spectrometry after derivatization with *p*-(hydroxymercuri)benzoate. Journal of Agricultural and Food Chemistry. 2010;**58**:1462-1468. DOI: 10.1021/jf903485k

[76] Prinsen HCMT, Schiebergen-Bronkhorst BGM, Roeleveld MW, Jan JJM, Sain-van Velden MGM, Visser G, van Hasselt PM, Verhoeven-Duif NM. Rapid quantification of underivatized amino acids in plasma by hydrophilic interaction liquid chromatography (HILIC) coupled with tandem mass-spectrometry. Journal of Inherited Metabolic Disease. 2016;**39**:651-660. DOI: 10.1007/s10545-016-9935-z

Homocysteine in Pathology

Chapter 3

Is Homocysteine a Marker or a Risk Factor: A Question Still Waits for an Answer

Cristiana Filip, Elena Albu, Hurjui Ion, Catalina Filip,
Cuciureanu Magda, Radu Florin Popa,
Demetra Gabriela Socolov, Ovidiu Alexa and
Alexandru Filip

Additional information is available at the end of the chapter

http://dx.doi.org/10.5772/intechopen.81799

Abstract

Homocysteine, a non-proteinogenic sulfur-containing amino acid, was discovered in 1932, and 30 years passed until, in 1969, for the first time, its involvement in pathology was reported. It was only in the last two decades that homocysteine has become a subject of scientific interest and has begun to be intensively studied. A large number of scientists consider homocysteine as an independent risk factor particularly for cardiovascular disease, while others indicate homocysteine as a marker of this disease. Both sides bring scientific arguments for their opinions, yet the dilemma of homocysteine characterization still persists. Although the reported studies do not lead to a unique answer, it is generally accepted that homocysteine is associated with vascular dysfunction. Numerous scientific data show that the link between homocysteine and inflammation is achieved via the reactive oxygen species (ROS) pathway. The latest data indicate hydrogen peroxide as a possible messenger in cellular signaling in physiological or pathological processes and present the consequences of disturbing the oxidation-reducing balance. In this chapter, we present the latest scientific evidences gathered from the literature for both hypotheses regarding homocysteine involvement in pathology, and we propose a possible mechanism of action for homocysteine, based on our preliminary (yet unpublished) work.

Keywords: hyperhomocysteinemia, ROS, inflammation, cell signaling, protein-tyrosine phosphatases

1. Introduction

Homocysteine (Hcy) is a non-proteinogenic amino acid that is formed in the human body in methionine metabolism. Although not forming proteins, homocysteine participates in major processes such as transmethylation, cysteine (Cys) formation, transsulfuration, etc. In the transmethylation process, homocysteine is an intermediate that allows the formation of compounds with a major metabolic role such as adrenaline, lecithin, creatine, etc. Cysteine formation, via homocysteine, is a very important process because Cys is a vital amino acid to stabilize the spatial conformations of proteins, to form the most important antioxidant agent in the body named glutathione, or to detoxify harmful compounds.

Over the past 40 years, homocysteine has come to the clinicians' attention because its high levels in blood have been associated with high risk of mortality and morbidity in many illnesses, particularly cardiovascular diseases. Patients with high levels of Hcy, also called hyperhomocysteinemia (HHcy), develop thromboembolism, premature atherosclerosis, mental retardation, bone fragility, eyes disease, and even miscarriage.

It is obvious that Hcy is related to the pathological phenomenon but the way it intervenes has not yet been elucidated. Moreover, there are researchers who believe that homocysteine indicates an already altered state [1] while others consider it a factor triggering the alteration of some functions [2]. Both opinions are based on scientific arguments, and although the debate continues, most researchers agree that there is an unquestionable link between homocysteine and vascular endothelial dysfunction [3–5]. Endothelial dysfunction may have several causes, but the major cause is inflammation. Inflammation is the vital process by which organisms respond to aggression. In the inflammatory process, a large number of pathways are activated to remove aggression and restore homeostasis [6–8]. Complex structures such as cells, proteins, but also small molecules such as reactive species, that are capable of rapidly signaling changes in homeostasis, are involved in this process. The activities of these structures need to be coordinated, and the latest data indicates that the inflammasome is responsible for this task. Recent data have found links between Hcy activity and inflammation [9]. In this chapter we present these new data that connect Hcy, inflammation, cell signaling, and reactive species.

As a conclusion, current data indicates Hcy as an amino acid that certainly plays a role in pathology, a role that needs to be elucidated.

2. Homocysteine metabolism

A short presentation of the homocysteine metabolism indicates two major pathways of transformation: the transmethylation pathway and the transsulfuration pathway (**Figure 1**).

Transmethylation pathway converts Hcy to methionine through a chain of reaction that involve the participation of methylenetetrahydrofolate reductase (MTHFR), folic acid, vitamin B12, and methionine synthase (MS).

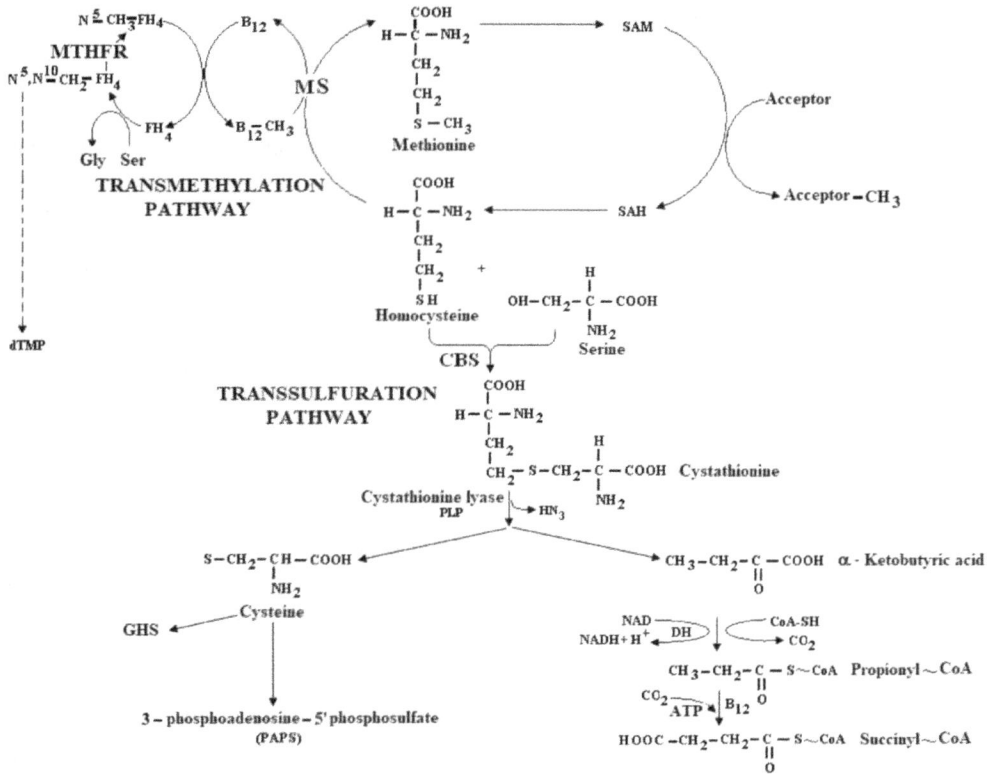

Figure 1. Main pathways of homocysteine transformation.

Transsulfuration pathway converts Hcy to cystathionine in the presence of the cystathionine beta-synthase (CBS) and vitamin B6. **Figure 1** highlights the role of tetrahydrofolate (FH4), the active form of folic acid, B12, and pyridoxal phosphate (PLP), the active form of vitamin B6 in the Hcy metabolism. A minor pathway, not shown in this figure, uses betaine to convert homocysteine to methionine.

The general methionine/homocysteine metabolism highlights the two major causes that generate HHcy: first, the enzymatic deficiencies of the enzymes acting in Hcy metabolization and, second, the nutritional deficiencies in vitamin cofactors. This last observation is the base of the therapeutic approaches that uses vitamin administration in order to decrease the homocysteine levels.

The normal concentration of homocysteine in human blood is 5–15 μM. HHcy is classified according to clinical consequences as being moderate at 16–30 μM, intermediary at 31–100 μM, and severe above 100 μM [10]. HHcy caused by the lack of vitamins is not commonly found in medical practice and it is easy to cure. The most common cause of HHcy is the enzymatic defect of different enzymes acting in this metabolism.

3. Homocysteine in pathology

3.1. Cardiovascular diseases

Currently, it is widely accepted that levels of Hcy, even at concentrations slightly higher than normal, are related to the risk of cardiovascular disease. Clinical studies indicate that a 5 µM increase in Hcy levels is equivalent to a 20 mg/dL increase in blood cholesterol [11, 12], which virtually doubles the cardiovascular risk. This suggests that between levels of Hcy and atherosclerosis there is a better correlation than between the cholesterol levels and atherosclerosis [13, 14]. However recent data [2, 15] show that a surprising 30% of cardiovascular mortality occurs in patients who do not present conventional risk factors as high LDL, hypertension, smoking, or obesity. This raises the question whether Hcy is an independent risk factor or it is a marker of a lesion process.

3.2. Diabetes

Hyperhomocysteinemia is considered a higher risk for patients with diabetes than nondiabetic patients. An exponential increase in vital risk has been demonstrated in patients presenting HHcy associated to diabetes [16–18]. The increase in Hcy levels noticed in diabetes is believed to be due to the degree of diabetes-induced nephropathy [19–21]. Thus, high levels of Hcy are found in kidney failure. This data suggest more for a marker role of homocysteine rather than a risk factor.

3.3. Neurological diseases

Seshadri [22] has shown that HHcy is associated with Alzheimer's disease and that it doubles the risk of developing the disease in patients with elevated levels of homocysteine as compared to those with normal levels. Although the mechanism that links Hcy to Alzheimer's is unknown, it is supposed that HHcy toxicity to neuronal cells is caused by possible neuronal damage following excessive stimulation caused as result of chronic central nervous system ischemia [23–25].

3.4. Bone fragility

Increased levels of homocysteine were correlated with increased risk of bone fractures in the elderly [26–31]. It seems that Hcy does not affect bone density but rather affects the structure of collagen by interfering in the transversal linkages between the collagen fibers. Thus, Hcy intervenes in tissue fortification showing more a risk factor role.

3.5. Miscarriage

Research studies notify that HHcy can be generated by the specific mutation in MTHFR. This inherited deficiency lead to a 3.3-fold increase in the risk of miscarriage in a sample group of 185 Caucasian women [32, 33]. Literature also specifies that associations between MTHFR C667T mutations to factor V Leiden and prothrombin gene mutations were identified in patients having recurrent miscarriages [34].

4. Homocysteine involvement in the endothelial function

The presented data show that in high concentration Hcy certainly plays a role in pathology. A large number of recent studies indicate that Hcy is an independent risk factor in cardiovascular disease [2, 35]. However, other studies indicate Hcy as a marker of this disease [1]. Although the reported studies do not lead to a unique answer regarding homocysteine role, it is generally agreed that homocysteine is connected to the vascular dysfunction. As a consequence, the investigation of HHcy leads to the investigation of endothelial dysfunction. Normal endothelial function consists in maintaining the vascular relaxation and the anticoagulant status. Any aggression on the endothelial homeostasis leads to changes in vascular morphology, tonicity, coagulability, etc. The intensity and time span of aggression determine the transition from a normal to a pathogenic transformation.

4.1. Endothelial dysfunction

Vascular endothelium modulates vascular tonicity by secreting a large group of vasoactive molecules such as vasodilators (e.g., NO, prostacyclin) and vasoconstrictors (e.g., endothelin, thromboxane). The ratio of these compounds showing antagonist action dictates the final vascular tonicity, and under pathological conditions, additional stimulants (mediators of inflammation) cause severe changes in vascular behavior.

Nitric oxide (NO) a natural free radical is synthesized by nitric oxide synthases (NOS) from L-arginine by many types of cells including the endothelial cells. Nitric oxide that is synthesized by endothelial nitric oxide synthase (eNOS) promotes vasodilatation; inhibits platelet activation, adhesion, and aggregation; prevents smooth muscle proliferation; and modulates endothelial-leucocytes interaction [36]. Homocysteine diminishes NO bioavailability through various processes that are, at least partially, based on oxidative mechanisms. The current literature presents three mechanisms proposed to explain the decrease in NO bioavailability in the presence of elevated levels of Hcy. The first mechanism indicates that Hcy reacts with nitric oxide to form S-nitroso-homocysteine [36, 37]. The second one considers that NO bioavailability is blocked by sequestration following reactions with other radical species. NO is trapped by superoxide to form peroxynitrite, thus being inactivated [38, 39]. The third mechanism assumes that NO synthesis is decreased by NO-synthase inhibition by asymmetric dimethylarginine (ADMA), a potent inhibitor of the enzyme produced by the degradation of methylated proteins [40]. Increased ADMA concentration was identified in an HHcy status [41]. These mechanisms are found widely presented in our previous work [42].

Eicosanoids represent a group of compounds directly involved in vascular function. They act as paracrine hormones and mediate the inflammatory response. This group includes prostacyclin (PGI2), a compound with vasodilating activity, and thromboxane TXA2, a compound with vasoconstrictive activity. Prostacyclin or prostaglandin PGI2, produced by epithelial cells, prevents platelet aggregation, decreases proliferation of smooth muscle cells, decreases pro-inflammatory cytokines (↓IL-1 and IL6), and exerts antimitogenic activity (↓VEGF and TGF-β). On contrary TXA2 promote the thrombosis and vascular constriction. In the chain of reactions that generates eicosanoids, some are of the oxidative type so they generate reactive species. Thus, the balance between these paracrine hormones is very important for the vascular homeostasis. Research data show that HHcy is considered as a factor that prevents vasodilation, promotes vasoconstriction, and increases the risk of thrombosis, thus inducing vascular injuries [43]. In vitro studies have demonstrated that HHcy induces the release of arachidonic acid, precursor of eicosanoids, including TXA2 [44].

Endothelins are vasoconstricting peptides mainly produced by the endothelium. They constrict blood vessel promoting high blood pressure. In addition to its vasoconstrictor effects, isoform endothelin-1 (ET-1) influences cell growth, thus being involved in atherosclerosis. Epithelial cells regulate ET-1 levels in response to hypoxia, oxidized species of LDL, or pro-inflammatory cytokines. Endothelins (ET-1, ET-2, ET-3) act on two receptors that have different locations and whose activation triggers different effects: vasoconstrictive effect through ET_A receptors located in smooth muscle cells [45] and vasodilation and NO release through ET_B receptors located on endothelial cells. Recent data show that HHcy results in the upregulation of ET_A receptor expression and high blood pressure in rats [46] while decreasing ET-1 production in endothelial cells, thus impairing NO and prostacyclin production and consequently the vasodilatation [47]. Thus, HHcy disturbs the ratio between vasodilators and vasoconstrictors promoting endothelial dysfunction [48].

5. Homocysteine mechanism of action

In the endothelial dysfunction, the inflammation process is a key step, and the reactive species are present at the site of inflammation, playing multiple roles, including defense, annihilation, or cellular signaling. In this chain of events, HHcy interferes somewhere with the endothelial normal function. There are several generally accepted mechanisms for Hcy-dependent endothelial dysfunction: *reactive oxygen species* [49], *inflammatory response* [50], or *thrombotic phenomenon* [51]. These mechanisms will be presented below along with scientific evidence for each of them.

5.1. Hyperhomocysteinemia involvement in oxidative stress

Numerous researches point ROS as the potential mediators for the effects of HHcy. Generation of reactive species is considered to trigger a cascade of events leading to release of pro-inflammatory cytokines, activation of adhesion molecules, generation of intracellular messengers that activate intracellular enzymes, and cellular responses including gene activation/repression [52–54]. Many studies demonstrate that HHcy generates reactive species directly or through autoxidation [55, 56]. ROS species found in HHcy was indirectly assessed through the measurement of antioxidative enzyme activity [57–59]. In our previous work, we have found that HHcy triggers the generation of hydrogen peroxide and that high levels of homocysteine experimentally induced (by methionine loading in rat) diminish more the total antioxidant capacity inside the erythrocytes rather than in plasma [60, 61].

5.2. Hyperhomocysteinemia involvement in inflammation

Recent studies [7, 8] had advanced the idea that Hcy triggers vascular damage by promoting an inflammatory response followed by immediate effects on the vascular wall or by delayed effects on proteins and DNA structures. The inflammatory phenomenon represents the vascular tissue response to lesion agents (chemical/physical or biological) [6]. The inflammatory response consists in two actions: removal of the lesion agent and initiation of the healing process. The acute inflammation predominates the local vascular response characterized by the presence of fast-acting and low half-life components (leucocytes). In the chronic inflammation, there is a progressive change in the types of cells present at the lesion site, characterized by the dominant presence of macrophages. The crucial phase is the destruction of pathogens. This phase takes place in monocytes/macrophages and neutrophils in the respiratory burst where the reactive oxygen species are generated. ROS are as damaging to pathogens as they are to the host's tissue. Consequently, chronic inflammation is accompanied by tissue destruction. Macrophages/neutrophils are not the site for respiratory burst only, but they also secret and/or trigger the secretion of specific compounds such as cytokines. The discovery of interleukins had introduced the concept of systemic inflammation. This type of inflammation is characterized by the fact that tissue destruction is not limited to a certain tissue but involves endothelium and other organs also. In systemic inflammation, elevated levels of chemical mediators such as interleukins (IL-6, IL-8, and TNFα) are associated with atherosclerosis and diabetes [62–64]. Recently, it has been found that HHcy is associated to inflammatory markers IL-6 and TNFα [65–68].

The cells of the innate immune system continually survey the extracellular environment in order to detect the "danger" signal. To achieve this function, immune cells develop receptors that act as sensors for the "invaders." Following the foreign detection, a group of actions must be initiated and coordinated, task being undertaken by the inflammasome. Inflammasomes are key signaling platforms that act as a checkpoint that controls and regulates the inflammatory response. It consists of multi-protein complexes that assemble by pattern-recognition receptors after the detection of a "danger "signal in the cytosol of the host cell. The protein association represents the activation stage of the inflammasome that triggers the signal of inflammation which is the caspase 1 and caspase 11 activation. Activated caspases initiate the highly pro-inflammatory cytokines' interleukin-1β (IL-1β) and IL-18 production, and finally an inflammatory form of cell death termed pyroptosis is triggered. The intracellular control of the inflammasome assembly is exerted via ion fluxes, free radicals, and autophagy. Latest data indicate the inflammasome activation as a possible mechanism for homocysteine involvement in inflammation and in programmed cell death in endothelial cells [69]. Current literature also demonstrates that the activation of inflammasomes (NLRP3 complex) represent a key step in HHcy-aggravated atherosclerosis [9].

5.3. Hyperhomocysteinemia involvement in thrombogenesis

HHcy promotes thrombosis by a mechanism that integrates the already presented processes of oxidation and decreases the NO bioavailability with the modification of some specific proteins acting in the coagulation and fibrinolysis pathway. Literatures show that homocysteine initiates structural modifications of these proteins, modifications that will impair their normal functions. Such proteins include the tissue plasminogen activator (tPA), atherogenic factor lipoprotein(a) (Lp(a)), the complex thrombomodulin-thrombin, and DNA proteins.

The tPA is a serine protease that converts plasminogen to fibrinolytic protein plasmin. Hcy forms disulfide bridge with annexin II (an important receptor for tissue plasminogen activator in endothelium), thus blocking tPA binding to this protein. As a result, tPA activity is impaired, plasmin generation is diminished, and fibrinolysis activity is decreased [70].

Activation of plasminogen depends on the binding of fibrin as a cofactor. Lipoprotein (a) is an atherogenic lipoprotein which competitively binds to fibrin, thus preventing activation of plasminogen. Hcy favors lipoprotein-a binding to fibrin, which ultimately leads to decreased fibrinolysis [71]. HHcy added to a dyslipidemia profile results in increased risk of thrombosis.

Protein C is another serine protease present in blood as zymogen. Upon activation it exerts important role in anticoagulation, inflammation, and also cell death. The complex thrombomodulin-thrombin activates protein C, thus inhibiting the thrombotic process. Hcy impairs the complex thrombomodulin-thrombin activity by forming disulfide bridges with both thrombomodulin and protein C. As a consequence, the thrombotic process is promoted [72]. These mechanisms are found widely presented in our previous work [42].

5.4. Hyperhomocysteinemia involvement in cellular signaling

The survival of the cell is by default linked to its ability to remove any type of aggression/lesion and to restore the initial healthy structure. In this process, cells develop a network of systems that is capable to communicate, to mobilize defense/healing structures, or to memorize information about the type of aggression. In this process, complex structures and small molecules are equally involved, together being able to signal any changes in homeostasis. Reactive species of oxygen and nitrogen as well as active peptides (cytokines) produced at the site of inflammation by neutrophils or monocytes/macrophages are small molecules capable of rapid signaling. They promote vascular changes and open the inter-endothelial junctions thus allowing the migration of inflammatory cells across the endothelial barrier. All the activities related to inflammatory response are coordinated by chemical signaling through reactive species signals or active peptides (cytokine) [73].

The link between reactive species and inflammation is now well documented. On the other hand, current data associate Hcy with both inflammation and reactive species. The factor that puts together all these components is not fully elucidated. Over the past two decades, many scientific evidences show that ROS serve in physiological as well as pathological processes [74, 75]. Normal levels of reactive species act as signaling molecules to regulate biological and physiological processes, while their accumulation is strongly associated with oxidative stress [76]. Current scientific data indicate that among reactive oxygen species hydrogen peroxide is the most likely secondary messenger [77]. Early data had signaled that exogenously added H_2O_2 could mimic growth factor activity and that the growth factors could stimulate the endogenous production of H_2O_2 within cells. [78–80]. A major role in cell signaling that promotes cell proliferation, nutrient uptake, and cell survival is realized by the activation of the protein-tyrosine kinases class which includes both tyrosine kinases (Src, Ras, JAK2, Pyk2, PI3K) and mitogen-activated protein kinases (MAPK) (**Figure 2**).

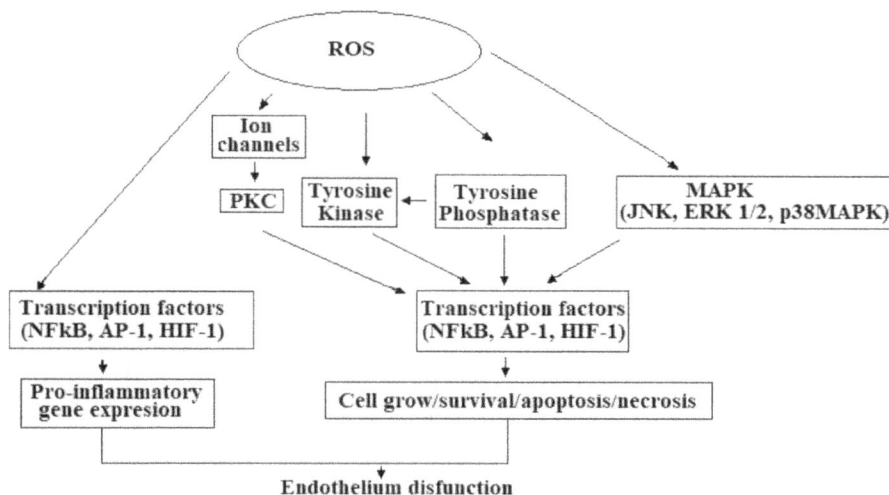

Figure 2. General signal pathway activated by ROS (modified from [81]), PKC = protein kinase, MAPK = mitogen-activated protein, JNK = c-Jun N-terminal kinases, ERK = extracellular signal-regulated kinases, NFκB = nuclear factor κB, AP-1 = activator protein-1, HIF-1 = hypoxia-inducible factor-1 C [42]. More details about the cellular response in ROS and other radical and nonradical species attack on oxidative events can be found in [82–84].

These signal transduction pathways use receptors with intrinsic tyrosine kinase activity (RTK) which leads to the phosphorylation of specific tyrosine residues located on tyrosine kinase proteins. Literatures show that hydrogen peroxide is required for optimal activation of protein-tyrosine kinases [85]. In the same time, hydrogen peroxide transiently inhibit protein-tyrosine phosphatases (PTPs) through the reversible oxidization of their catalytic cysteine [86], thus suppressing protein-tyrosine kinases dephosphorylation [87]. Thus, the activity of MAPK kinases is negatively regulated by protein-tyrosine phosphatases as depicted in **Figure 3**.

Protein-tyrosine phosphatases are specific proteins that contain cysteine residues at their active site. These enzymes remove a phosphate group attached to a tyrosine residue (such in MAP kinases), using a cysteinyl-phosphate enzyme intermediate. Latest literature data [88,89] show that the activity of protein-tyrosine phosphatases is regulated by the reversible oxidation of cysteine residues. In the reversible oxidation, the PTPs activity results in temporarily dampening of mitogenic signaling [84, 90]. Protein-tyrosine phosphatases can suffer an irreversible oxidation to their thiol groups, in the presence of high H_2O_2 levels, [91]. As a result, their function is blocked and the mitogen signal remains continuously activated (**Figure 3**).

Cysteine is unique among the amino acids because it is the only proteinogenic amino acid containing a free SH group. The mechanism of redox signaling involves reversible H_2O_2-mediated oxidation of cysteine residues within proteins [92]. During redox signaling low/normal concentration of H_2O_2 (nM range) oxidizes the thiol group of cysteine residues to sulfenic form (Cys-SOH). As the concentration of H_2O_2 gradually increases, the sulfenic form

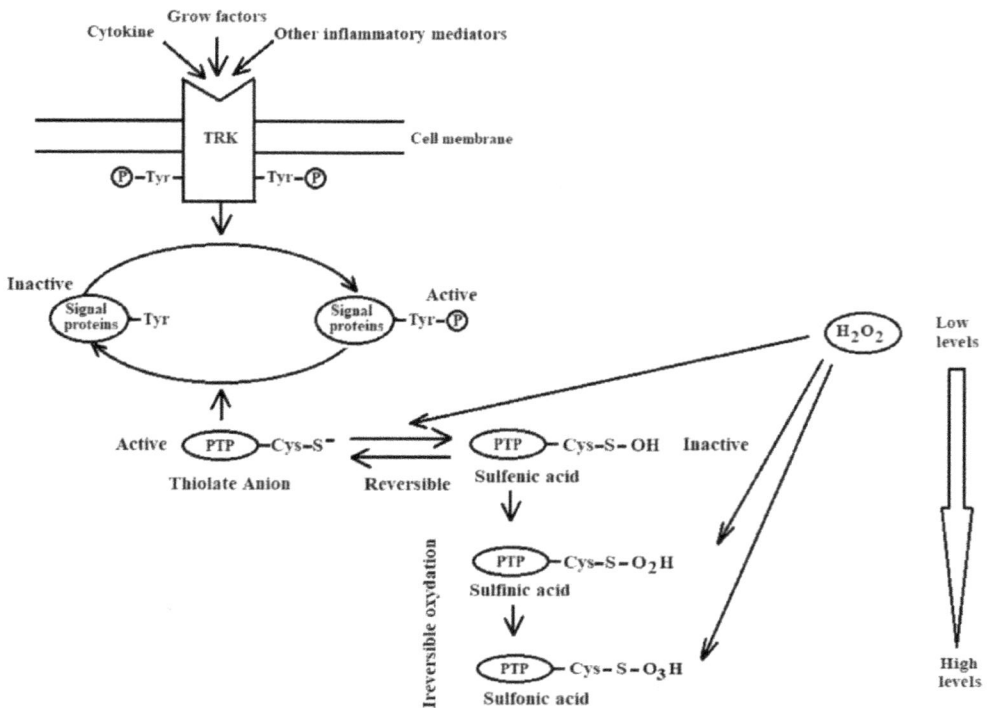

Figure 3. Hydrogen peroxide role in protein-tyrosine kinases regulation. In normal/low concentration, H_2O_2 regulates PTPs activity by promoting the reversible oxidation of the Cys residues. At high concentration of H_2O_2, PTPs becomes irreversibly inactive and, as a consequence, tyrosine kinase proteins involved in cell proliferation (MAPK) remain blocked on active form. TRK = receptors with intrinsic tyrosine kinase activity; and PTP = proteon-tyrosine phosphatases.

transforms to sulfinic (SO_2H) and sulfonic (SO_3H) forms, respectively. Unlike sulfenic modifications, sulfinic and sulfonic are irreversible transformations. As a consequence, high levels of H_2O_2 can trigger the irreversible oxidation of cysteine group.

Considering the above data, it is possible that Hcy, a H_2O_2 generator according to scientific data, may interfere in this signaling process promoting mitogenic activity.

Moreover, Hcy is very similar in structure to cysteine. Like cysteine, Hcy is an amino acid containing a free SH group. This makes possible the occurrence of disulfide bridges between the two amino acids similar to those existing between cysteine residues in some particular concentration of hydrogen peroxide. In our opinion (preliminary work, unpublished data), this may be a possible mechanism of homocysteine involvement in cell signaling that must be investigated (**Figure 4**).

All the scientific evidence presented above suggest Hcy as a risk factor for the vascular/endothelial dysfunction.

Instead some scientists investigate Hcy from the opposite point of view [93] and consider HHcy as a marker of an already altered vascular state rather than a risk factor. These authors

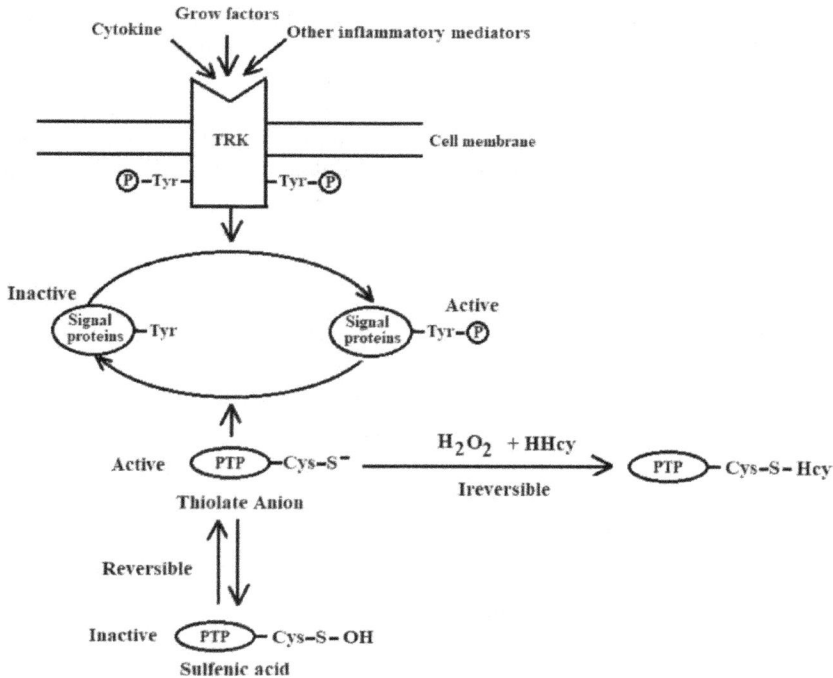

Figure 4. Possible mechanism for hyperhomocysteinemia to intercept the protein-tyrosine phosphatase regulation through disulfide bridge formation. TRK = receptors with intrinsic tyrosine kinase activity; PTP = proteon-tyrosine phosphatases; and HHcy = hyperhomocysteinemia.

consider that hypertension and atherosclerosis reach the stage where kidney function is severally impaired and Hcy removal is diminished and, consequently, its concentration rises in the blood. Atherosclerosis and hypertension are silent diseases that develop years before a vascular event occurs. The disease is accompanied by a silent decline in renal function and, as a consequence, total clearance including that of homocysteine diminishes. Thus, vascular disease contributes to the elevation of circulating Hcy as result of the progressive decline in renal function, and HHcy in fact reflects the severity of atherosclerosis. Thus, HHcy becomes a signal that the atherosclerotic disease reaches an irreversible stage.

Regardless of the classification of homocysteine as a risk factor or marker, its involvement in pathology is certain, and its role needs to be elucidated.

6. Conclusion

The study of homocysteine began when its association with cardiovascular disease was discovered. Further studies revealed its association with vascular dysfunction, and then Hcy was linked to the inflammatory phenomenon. Recently, as studies advanced, the homocysteine involvement in inflammation has been identified. The inflammatory process in turn is related to the activity of reactive species, and recent data indicate protein-tyrosine phosphatases as key factors in regulating intracellular signaling pathways. These proteins allow regulation because they can undergo reversible oxidation phenomena due to the presence in their structure of cysteine residues bearing SH groups. The structural similarity of Cys with homocysteine draws attention to the possibility that Hcy may interfere with cysteine functions. In conclusion, the recent association of Hcy with both inflammation and the reactive species involved in cellular signaling indicates that homocysteine remains a topic of interest and attention in current research. It is obvious that HHcy is an issue of interest in contemporary medicine.

Author details

Cristiana Filip[1]*, Elena Albu[2], Hurjui Ion[3], Catalina Filip[4], Cuciureanu Magda[2], Radu Florin Popa[4], Demetra Gabriela Socolov[5], Ovidiu Alexa[6] and Alexandru Filip[6]

*Address all correspondence to: cfilip2000@yahoo.com

1 Department of Biochemistry, University of Medicine and Pharmacy "Grigore T. Popa", Iasi, Romania

2 Department of Pharmacology, University of Medicine and Pharmacy "Grigore T. Popa", Iasi, Romania

3 Department of Biophysics, University of Medicine and Pharmacy "Grigore T. Popa", Iasi, Romania

4 Department of Vascular Surgery, University of Medicine and Pharmacy "Grigore T. Popa", Iasi, Romania

5 Department of Obstetrics and Gynecology, University of Medicine and Pharmacy "Grigore T. Popa", Iasi, Romania

6 Department of Orthopedics and Traumatology, University of Medicine and Pharmacy "Grigore T. Popa", Iasi, Romania

References

[1]   Zhang S, Yong-Yi B, Luo LM, Xiao WK, Wu HM, Ye P. Association between serum homocysteine and arterial stiffness in elderly: A community-based study. Journal of Geriatric Cardiology. 2014;**11**(1):32-38

[2]   Salemi G, Gueli MC, Vitale F, et al. Blood lipids, homocysteine, stress factor and vitamins in clinically stable multiple sclerosis patients. Lipids in Health and Disease. 2010;**9**(1):19

[3]   Hassan A, Hunt BJ, O'Sullivan M, Bell R, D'Souza R, Jeffery S, et al. Homocysteine is a risk factor for cerebral small vessel disease, acting via endothelial dysfunction. Brain. 2004;**127**(1):212-219

[4] Pushpakumar S, Kundu S, Sen Y. Endothelial dysfunction: The link between homocysteine and hydrogen sulfide. Current Medicinal Chemistry. 2014;21(32):3662-3672

[5] Lai WK, Kan MY. Homocysteine-induced endothelial dysfunction. Annals of Nutrition & Metabolism. 2015;67(1):1-12

[6] Ferrero-Miliani L, Nielsen OH, Andersen PS, Girardin SE. Chronic inflammation: Importance of NOD2 and NALP3 in interleukin-1beta generation. Clinical and Experimental Immunology. 2007;147(2):227-235

[7] Shastry S, James LR. Homocysteine-induced macrophage inflammatory protein-2 production by glomerular mesangial cells is mediated by PI3 kinase and p38 MAPK. Journal of Inflammation. 2009;6:27. DOI: 10.1186/1476-9255-6-27

[8] Zhang X, Chen S, Li L, Wang Q, Le W. Folic acid protects motor neurons against the increased homocysteine, inflammation and apoptosis in SOD1^{G93A} transgenic mice. Europharmacology. 2008;54(7):1112-1119

[9] Wang R, Wang I, Mu N, Lou X, Li W, Chen Y, et al. Activation of NLRP3 inflammasomes contributes to hyperhomocysteinemia-aggravated inflammation and atherosclerosis in apoE-deficient mice. Laboratory Investigation. 2017;97(8):922-934

[10] Filip C, Albu E, Lupascu D, Filip N. The influence of a new rutin derivative in an experimental model of induced hyperhomocysteinemia in rats. Farmacia. 2017;65(4):596-599

[11] Hadi HA, Carr CS, Al Suwaidi J. Endothelial dysfunction: Cardiovascular risk factors, therapy, and outcome. Vascular Health and Risk Management. 2005;1(3):183-198

[12] Candido R, Zanetti M, Current p. Diabetic vascular disease: From endothelial dysfunction to atherosclerosis. Italian Heart Journal. 2005;6(9):703-720

[13] Saposnik G, Ray JG, Sheridan P, McQeen M, Lonn E. Homocysteine-lowering therapy and stroke risk, severity and disability: Additional findings from HOPE 2 trial. Stroke. 2009;40(4):1365-1372

[14] Humphrey LL, Fu R, Rogers K, Freeman M, Helfand M. Homocysteine level and coronary disease: A systematic review and meta-analysis. Mayo Clinic Proceedings. 2008 Nov;83(11):1203-1212

[15] Melichar B, Kalabova H, Krcmova L, et al. Serum homocysteine, cholesterol, alpha-tocopherol, glycosylated hemoglobin and inflammatory response during therapy with bevacizumab, oxaliplatin, 5-fluorouracil and leucovorin. Anticancer Research. 2009;29(11):4813-4820

[16] Shukla N, Angelini GD, Jeremy JY. The administration of folic acid reduces intravascular oxidative stress in diabetic rabbits. Metabolism. 2008;57(6):774-781

[17] Terzic–Avdagic. Correlation of coronary disease in patients with diabetes mellitus type 2. Journal of Medical Archives. 2009;63(4):191-193

[18] Snoki K, Iwase M, Sasaki N, Ohdo S, Higuchi S, Matsuyama N, et al. Relations of lysophosphatidylcholine in low-density lipoprotein with serum lipoprotein-associated

phospholipase A2, paraoxonase and homocysteine thiolactonase activities in patients with type 2 diabetes mellitus. Diabetes Research and Clinical Practice. 2009;**86**(2):117-123

[19] Sen U, Rodriguez WE, Tyagi N, Kumar M, Kundu S, Tyagi SC. Ciglitazone a PPAR γ agonist, ameliorate diabetic nephropathy in part through homocysteine clearance. American Journal of Physiology. Endocrinology and Metabolism. 2008;**295**:E1205-E1212

[20] Wei J, Qiang Y, Yong-ping L, Hui-ming W, Xiang-qun H, Shu-qioa Y, et al. Serum metrix metalloproteinase-9 combined with homocysteine, IL-6, TNF-α, CRP, HbA1c and lipid profile in the incipient diabetic nephropathy with or without macrovascular diseases. Journal of Medical Colleges of PLA. 2007;**22**(2):111-114

[21] Friedman AN, Hunsicker LG, Selhub J, Bostom AG. Total plasma homocysteine and arteriosclerotic outcomes in type 2 diabetes with nephropathy. Journal of the American Society of Nephrology. 2005;**16**:3397-3402

[22] Sudha Seshadri MD, Philip A, Wolf MD, Beiser AS, Selhub J, Au R, et al. Association of plasma total homocysteine levels with subclinical brain injury. Archives of Neurology. 2008;**65**(5):642-649

[23] Vidal J-S, Dufouil C, Ducros V, Tzourio C. Homocysteine, folate and cognition in a large community-based sample of elderly people–The 3C Dijon study. Neuroepidemiology. 2008;**30**:207-214

[24] Zylberstein DE, Skoog I, Björkelund C, Guo X, Hultén B, Andreasson L-A, et al. Homocysteine levels and lacunar brain infarcts in elderly women: The prospective population study of women in Gothenburg. Journal of the American Geriatrics Society. 2008;**56**(6):1087-1091

[25] David Smith A, Refsum H, Bottiglieri T, Fenech M, Hoosmand B, McCaddon A, et al. Homocysteine and dementia: An international consensus statement. Journal of Alzheimer's Disease. 2018;**62**(2):561-570

[26] Sato Y, Honda Y, Iwamoto J, Kanoko T, Satoh K. Effect of folate and mecobalamin on hip fractures in patients with stroke: A randomized controlled trial. JAMA. 2005; **293**(9):1082-1088

[27] Rhew EY, Lee C, Eksarko P, Dyer AR, Tily H, Spies S, et al. Homocysteine, bone mineral density, and fracture risk over 2 years of followup in women with and without systemic lupus erythematosus. The Journal of Rheumatology. 2008;**35**(2):230-236

[28] Green TJ, McMahon JA, Skeaff CM, Williams SM, Whiting SJ. Lowering homocysteine with B vitamins has no effect on biomarkers of bone turnover in old persons: A 2-y randomized controlled trial. The American Journal of Clinical Nutrition. 2007;**85**:460-464

[29] Cagnacci A. Relation of folates, vitamin B12 and homocysteine to vertebral bone mineral density change in postmenopausal women. A five-year longitudinal evaluation. Bone. **42**(2):314-320

[30] Filip A, Filip N, Veliceasa B, Filip C, Alexa O. The relationship between homocysteine and fragility fractures–A systematic review. Annual Research & Review in Biology. **16**(5). ISSN: 2347-565X

[31] Filip N, Cojocaru E, Filip A, Veliceasa B, Alexa O. Reactive Oxygen Species (ROS) in living cells. In: InTech, editor. Chapter 4 Reactive Oxygen Species and Bone Fragility. Rijeka, Croatia: InTech; 2018. pp. 49-67

[32] Nelen WL, Steegers EA, Eskes TK, et al. Genetic risk factor for unexplained recurrent early pregnancy loss. Lancet. 1997;**350**:861

[33] Merviel P, Cabry R, Lourdel E, Lanta S, Amant C, Copin H, et al. Comparison of two preventive treatments for patient with recurrent miscarriages carrying C677T meth-ylenetetrahydrofolate *redu*ctase mutation: 5-year experience. Journal of International Medical Research. 2017;**45**(6):1720-1730

[34] Abdelsalam T, Karkour T, Elbordiny M, Shalaby D, Abouzeid ZS. Thrombophilia gene mutations in relation to recurrent miscarriage. International Journal of Reproduction, Contraception, Obstetrics and Gynecology. 2018;**7**:796-800

[35] Baszczuk A, Kopczynski Z. Hyperhomocysteinemia in patients with cardiovascular dis-ease. Postępy Higieny i Medycyny Doświadczalnej. 2014;**68**:579

[36] Thambyrajah J, Townend JN. Homocysteine and atherothrombosis-mechanism for injury. European Heart Journal. 2000;**21**:967-974

[37] Upchurch GR Jr, Welch GN, Loscalzo J. Homocysteine, EDRF, and endothelial function. The Journal of Nutrition. 1996;**126**(4 Suppl):1290S-4S.29

[38] Upchurch GR, Welch G, Fabian A, et al. Homocysteine decreases bioavailable nitric oxide by a mechanism involving glutathione peroxidase. The Journal of Biological Chemistry. 1997;**272**:17012-17017

[39] Welch GN, Loscalzo J. Homocysteine and atherothrombosis. The New England Journal of Medicine. 1998;**338**:1042-1050

[40] Zakrzewicz D, Eickelberg O. From arginine methylation to ADMA: A novel mechanism with therapeutic potential in chronic lung diseases. BMC Pulmonary Medicine. 2009;**9**:5

[41] Sydow K, Schwedhelm E, Arakawa N, Bode-Boger SM, Tsikas D, Hornig B, et al. ADMA and oxidative stress are responsible for endothelial dysfunction in hyperhomocystein-emia: Effects of L-arginine and B vitamins. Cardiovascular Research. 2003;**57**:244-252

[42] Cristiana F, Nina Z, Elena A. Blood cell–An overview of studies in hematology, In: InTech, editor. Homocysteine in Red Blood Cells Metabolism–Pharmacological Approaches. Rijeka, Croatia: InTech; 2012. pp. 31-68. ISBN 978-953-51-0753-8

[43] Ma Y, Peng D, Liu C, Huang C, Luo J. Serum high concentration of homocysteine and low levels of folic acid and vitamin B_{12} are significantly correlated with the categories of coronary artery disease. BMC Cardiovascular Disorders. 2017;**17**:37

[44] Leoncini G, Bruzzesse D, Signorello MG. Activation of p38 MAPKinase/cPLA2 path-way in homocysteine-treated platelets. Journal of Thrombosis and Hemostasis. 2005; **4**(1):209-216

[45] Hynynen MM, Khalil RA. The vascular endothelin system in hypertension-recent patents and discoveries. Recent Patents on Cardiovascular Drug Discovery. 2006;**1**(1):95-108

[46] Chen Y, Liu H, Wang X, Zhang H, Liu E, Su X. Homocysteine up-regulates endothelin type A receptor in vascular smooth muscle cell through SIRT1/ERK1/2 signaling pathway. Microvascular Research. 2017;**114**:34-40

[47] Demuth K, Atger VÂ, Borderie D, Benoit M-O, Sauvaget D, Lotersztajn S, et al. Homocysteine decreases endothelin-1 production by cultured human endothelial cells. European Journal of Biochemistry. 1999;**263**:367-376

[48] Salaets K, Schliessman J, Speiser R, Tran A-M, Wang E, Angerio DA. The role of endothelin-1 in atherosclerosis. Georgetown University Journal of Health Sciences. 2006;**3**(1). https://blogs.commons.georgetown.edu/journal-of-health-sciences/issues-2/previous-volumes/vol-3-no-1-march-2006/role-of-endothelin-1-in-atherosclerosis/

[49] Mangge H, Becker K, Fuchs D, Gostner JM. Antioxidants, inflammation and cardiovascular disease. World Journal of Cardiology. 2014;**6**(6):462-477

[50] Pang X, Liu J, Zhao J, Mao J, Zhang X, Feng L, et al. Homocysteine induces the expression of C–reactive protein via NMDAr-ROS-MAPK-NF-κB signal pathway in rat vascular smooth muscle cells. Atherosclerosis. 2014;**236**:73-81

[51] Xie R, Jia D, Gao C, Zhou J, Sui H, Wei X, et al. Homocysteine induces procoagulant activity of red blood cells via phosphatidylserine exposure and microparticles generation. Amino Acids. 2014;**46**:1997-2004. DOI: 10.1007/s00726-014-1755-6

[52] Sibrian-Vazquez M, Escobedo JO, Lim S, Samoei GK, Strongin RM. Homocystamides promote free-radical and oxidative damage to proteins. Proceedings of the National Academy of Sciences of the United States of America. 2010;**107**(2):551-554

[53] Papatheodorou L, Weiss N. Vascular oxidant stress and inflammation in hyperhomocysteinemia. Antioxidants & Redox Signaling. 2007;**9**:1941-1958

[54] Zou CG, Banerjee R. Homocysteine and redox signaling. Antioxidants & Redox Signaling. 2005;**7**:547-559

[55] Pang X, Liu J, Zhao J, Mao J, Zhang X, Feng L, et al. Homocysteine induces the expression of C–reactive protein via NMDAr-ROS-MAPK-NF-κB signal pathway in rat vascular smooth muscle cells. Atherosclerosis. 2014;**236**:73-816

[56] Starkebaum G, Harlan JM. Endothelial injury due to cooper-catalyzed hydrogen peroxide generation from homocysteine. The Journal of Clinical Investigation. 1986;**77**:1370-1376

[57] Filip C, Albu E, Zamosteanu N, Jerca L, Gheorghita N, Jaba IM, et al. Investigarea parametrilor stresului oxidativ in hiperhomocisteinemia provocata experimental la sobolan. Medicina Moderna. 2009;**XVI**(Suppl. 1):191-193

[58] Albu E, Filip C, Zamosteanu N, Jaba IM, Gheorghita N, Jerca L, et al. The influence on the experimental stress on the plasma level of homocysteine, in rat, therapeutics. Pharmacology and Clinical Toxicology. 2009;**XIII**(2):143-146

[59] Albu E, Filip C, Zamosteanu N, Dimitriu DC, Jaba IM, Gheorghita N, et al. Investigation of correlation stress-hyperhomocysteinemia. Therapeutics, Pharmacology and Clinical Toxicology. 2009;**XIII**(3):261-265

[60] Filip C, Albu E, Nina Zamosteanu M, Irina J, Silion M. Hyperhomocysteinemia's effect on antioxidant capacity on rats. Central European Journal of Medicine. 2010;**5**(5):620-626

[61] Albu E, Filip C, Zamosteanu N, Jaba IM, Linic IS, Sosa I. Hyperhomocysteinemia is an indicator of oxidant stress. Medical Hypotheses. 2012;**78**(4):554-555

[62] Stitzinger M. Lipids, inflammation and atherosclerosis, (2007), the digital repository of Leiden University, pdf, Hansson GK inflammation, atherosclerosis and coronary disease. The New England Journal of Medicine. (2005);**352**:0685-1695

[63] Libby P, Theroux P. Pathophysiology of coronary artery disease. Circulation. 2005; **111**:3481-3488

[64] Luis AJ. Atherosclerosis. Nature. 2000;**407**:233-241

[65] El Oudi M, Aouni Z, Mazigh C, Gazoueni E, Haouela H, Machghoul S. Homocysteine and markers of inflammation in acute coronary syndrome. Experimental and Clinical Cardiology. 2010;**15**(2):e25-e28

[66] Gori AM, Sofi F, Marcucci R, Abbate R. Association between homocysteine, vitamin B6 concentrations and inflammation. Clinical Chemistry and Laboratory Medicine. 2007; **45**(12):1728-1736

[67] Ganguly P, Alam SF. Role of homocysteine in the development of cardiovascular disease. Nutrition Journal. 2015;**14**:6

[68] Li T, Chen Y, Li J, Yang X, Zhang H, Qin X, Hu Y, Mo Z. Serum homocysteine concentration is significantly associated with inflammatory/immune factors. PLoS One. 2015;**10**(9)

[69] Xi H, Zhang Y, Xu Y, Yang WY, Jiang SX, Cheng X, et al. Caspase-1 inflammasome activation mediates homocysteine induced pyro-apoptosis in endothelial cells. Circulation Research. 2016;**118**(10):1526-1539

[70] Carmel R, Jacobsen DW. Homocysteine in Health and Disease. Cambridge University Press; 2001. ISBN: 0 521 65319 3

[71] Harpel PC, Zhang X. Borth, homocysteine and hemostasis: Pathogenic mechanism predisposing to thrombosis. Nutrition. 1996;**126**(4 Suppl):1285S-1289S

[72] Lentzt SR, Evan Sadler J. Inhibition of thrombomodulin surface expression and protein C activation by the thrombogenic agent homocysteine. The Journal of Clinical Investigation. 1991;**88**:1906-1914

[73] Mittal M, Siddiqui MR, Tran K, Reddy SP, Malik AB. Reactive oxygen species in inflammation and tissue injury. Antioxidants & Redox Signaling. 2014;**20**(7):1126-1167

[74] Schieber M, Chandel NS. ROS function in redox signaling and oxidative stress. Current Biology. 2014;**24**(10):R453-R462

[75] Forman HJ, Maiorino M, Ursini F. Signaling function of reactive oxygen species. Biochemistry. 2010;**49**(5):835-842

[76] Murphy MP. Mitochondrial thiols in antioxidant protection and redox signaling: Distinct roles for glutathionylation and other thiol modifications. Antioxidants & Redox Signaling. 2012;**16**:476-495

[77] Forman HJ, Maiorino M, Ursini F. Signaling function of reactive oxygen species. Biochemistry. 2010;**49**(5):835-842

[78] Czech MP. Differential effects of sulfhydryl reagents on activation and deactivation of the fat cell hexose transport system. The Journal of Biological Chemistry. 1976;**251**:1164-1170

[79] Mukherjee SP, Lane RH, Lynn WS. Endogenous hydrogen peroxide and peroxidative metabolism in adipocytes in response to insulin and sulfhydryl reagents. Biochemical Pharmacology. 1978;**27**:2589-2594

[80] Mukherjee SP, Mukherjee C. Similar activities of nerve growth factor and its homologue proinsulin in intracellular hydrogen peroxide production and metabolism in adipocytes. Trans-membrane signaling relative to insulin-mimicking cellular effects. Biochemical Pharmacology. 1982;**31**:3163-3172

[81] Bahorun T, Soobratte MA, Luximon-Ramma V, Aruoma OI. Free radicals and antioxidants in cardiovascular health and disease. Internet Journal of Medical Update. 2006;**1**(2):25-41

[82] Novo E, Parola M. Redox mechanisms in hepatic chronic wound healing and fibrogenesis. Fibrogenesis & Tissue Repair. 2008;**1**:58

[83] Martindale JL, Holbrook NJ. Cellular response to oxidative stress: Signaling for suicide and survival. Journal of Cellular Physiology. 2002;**192**(1):1-15

[84] Powers SK, Duarte J, Kavazis AN, Talbert EE. Reactive oxygen species are signaling molecules for skeletal muscle adaptation. Experimental Physiology. 2010;**95**:1-9

[85] Sun JP, Zhang ZY, Wang WQ. An overview of the protein tyrosine phosphatase superfamily. Current Topics in Medicinal Chemistry. 2003;**3**(7):739-748

[86] Winterbourn CC, Hampton MB. Thiol chemistry and specificity in redox signaling. Free Radical Biology & Medicine. 2008;**45**:549-561

[87] Carty NC, Xu J, Kurup P, Brouillette J, Goebel-Goody SM, Austin DR, et al. The tyrosine phosphatase STEP: Implications in schizophrenia and the molecular mechanism underlying antipsychotic medications. Translational Psychiatry. 2012;**2**(7):e137

[88] Finkel T. Signal transduction by reactive oxygen species. The Journal of Cell Biology. 2011;**194**(1):7-15

[89] Louro RO, Diaz-Moreno I. Redox Proteins in Super Complexes and Signalosomes. Boca Raton, FL: CRC Press; 2016. p. 338

[90] Kobayashi Y, Ito K, Kanda A, Tomoda K, Miller-Larsson A, Barnes PJ, et al. Protein tyrosine phosphatase PTP-RR regulates corticosteroid sensitivity. Respiratory Research. 2016;**17**:30

[91] Marino SM, Gladyshev VN, Marino SM, Gladyshev VN. Cysteine function governs its conservation and degeneration and restricts its utilization on protein surface. Journal of Molecular Biology. 2010;**404**:902-916

[92] Rhee S. Cell signaling. H_2O_2, a necessary evil for cell signaling. Science. 2006;**312**:1882-1883

[93] Brattström L, Wilcken DEL. Homocysteine and cardiovascular disease: Cause or effect? The American Journal of Clinical Nutrition. 2000;**72**(2):315-323

Chapter 4

How Homocysteine Modulates the Function of Osteoblasts and Osteocytes

Viji Vijayan and Sarika Gupta

Additional information is available at the end of the chapter

http://dx.doi.org/10.5772/intechopen.76398

Abstract

Over the years, numerous mechanisms have been identified through which homocysteine affects osteoblast functioning. These include alterations in collagen structure, epigenetic modifications and changes in RANKL-OPG production by osteoblasts. These mechanisms are reviewed in this chapter. We have also herein discussed how homocysteine affects osteocyte behavior. With onset of hyperhomocysteinemia induction of osteocyte specific genes particularly the mineralization genes like Dmp1 and Sost is facilitated producing untoward mineralization, osteocyte apoptosis, deviations from regular bone remodeling process and onset of targeted remodeling in bone. These modifications have immense effect on the overall mechanical stability of bone. Homocysteine thus represents an independent risk factor for bone fragility.

Keywords: homocysteine, osteoblast, osteocyte, sclerostin, dentine matrix protein1

1. Introduction

Bone remodelling is a process that occurs throughout life. This process occurs to replace old mineralized bone with new bone, preserve bone mass, mineral homeostasis, pH balance, repair microdamage, maintain glucose homeostasis and preserve male fertility. Bone remodeling is a highly co-ordinated process that requires the controlled activities of many systemic and local factors like calcitriol, parathyroid hormone, growth hormone, thyroid hormones, glucocorticoids, bone morphogenetic proteins, prostaglandins, sex hormones, various cytokines and the molecular triad comprising of OPG (osteoprotegerin), receptor activator of nuclear factor-κB ligand (RANKL) and receptor activator of nuclear factor-κB (RANK). The cells involved in the process are osteoblasts, osteoclasts, osteocytes, immune cells, megakaryocytes and osteomacs.

IntechOpen

With senescence, decreased production of sex hormones like estrogen and testosterone, susceptibility to genetic and environmental factors and life style modifications; the process of bone remodeling process gets hampered increasing the rate of bone resorption as compared to that of bone formation. Such deviations from normal bone remodeling process deplete the bone of its minerals like calcium and proteins like collagen affecting the overall mass and mechanical property of the bone, escalating the risk of bone fractures [1, 2].

Many metabolic substances also affect bone. One such factor is homocysteine. Since its discovery in 1932, homocysteine has remained an important aspect for research. Homocysteine is basically a metabolite of methionine metabolism that exists at a critical biochemical point in the methionine cycle from where it is used to synthesize cysteine and glutathione. When re-methylation and transsulfuration cycles in methionine cycle collapse owing to an enzyme or co-factor deficiency, homocysteine accumulate in blood resulting in a clinical condition called hyperhomocysteinemia (>15 micromol/L). The prevalence of hyperhomocysteinemia varies with geography, age, sex and ethnicity. Till date high level of methionine, deficiency of enzymes in methionine metabolism like cystathionine synthase (a pyridoxal phosphate dependent enzyme), methionine synthase (a folate and vitamin B12 dependent enzyme) and methylene-tetrahydrofolate reducatase, deficiency of vitamins like folate and vitamin B_{12} in diet (caused by losses of these sensitive vitamins by methods of food processing such as milling of grains, canning, extraction of sugars and oils, radiation and chemical additives), environmental elements, life-style habits, hormonal changes, drugs and diseases like cardiovascular, cancer and type 2 diabetes have been found to be causes for hyperhomocysteinemia.

The negative effect of homocysteine on the bone is well supported by the demonstrations of loss of bone physiology in experimental animals of hyperhomocysteinemia generated by administering a methionine-enriched diet (with low folate) as well in genetic models of enzyme deficiency [3]. This chapter will present the current findings on how hyperhomocysteinemia alters the functions of two types of bone cells—the osteoblast and the osteocyte.

1.1. How homocysteine affects osteoblast function?

Studies on the effect of homocysteine on bone forming osteoblasts have shown that homocysteine is different from a conventional oxidant and exerts its effects on cells via multiple modes. Over the years diverse mechanisms were identified by which homocysteine affects osteoblast functioning. These include alterations in collagen structure, epigenetic modifications and changes in RANKL-OPG production by osteoblasts. The first example to cite how homocysteine alters osteoblast machinery was a clinical study by Hermann et al. in 2005 [4]. The results of this study showed that a positive correlation occurs between hyperhomocysteinemia and circulating concentrations of osteocalcin, an osteoblast activity marker. In contrast to this finding was a report by Sakamoto et al. in the same year 2005 [5], which demonstrated that homocysteine, stimulates only osteopontin and has an attenuating effect on osteocalcin. The paper also revealed that homocysteine represents an independent risk factor for osteoporosis. In the subsequent years 2007–2008, clinical studies by Hermann et al. [6, 7] published the following: Accumulation of homocysteine caused by "reduction in co-factors of methionine metabolism like folate, vitamin B_{12} and vitamin B_6" do not cause any change in the activities of alkaline phosphatase, osteocalcin and pro-collagen type I N-terminal peptide (PINP) in serum. However such low concentrations of folate, vitamin B_{12} and vitamin B_6 are enough to produce a stimulatory effect on osteoclast activity. This study also rationalized the mechanistic role of low B-vitamin concentrations for bone degradation. The same research group also demonstrated how direct exposure of primary human osteoblasts to increasing concentrations of homocysteine stimulates cellular activity. This report brought about the awareness that homocysteine "not inhibits but alters" osteoblast function, one of the reasons why some of results of clinical and experimental studies were in disagreement with each other. In the subsequent years Thaler et al. [8–10] reported noteworthy mechanisms regarding how homocysteine affected the bone matrix. The authors showed that homocysteine altered collagen cross linking by inhibiting the expression of lysyl hydroxylase and lysyl oxidase, enzymes required for formation of stable bone matrix. Collagen cross linking in the bone is a post translational modification of collagen molecules that play integral role in tissue differentiation and render mechanical support to the bone. The authors revealed that homocysteine uncovers RGD motif (a tripeptide of Arg-Gly-Asp) in collagen by RelA protein activation. Collagens are important structural proteins that form the extracellular matrix and play important role in shaping and organizing a tissue and the major collagen found in the bone is type 1 collagen. When denatured, type 1 collagen unwinds its triple helical structure causing the exposure of RGD motifs in it. Such exposure is basically a mechanism by which signals are presented to cells for regulating cell behavior, promoting tissue repair and regeneration. But when exposed to homocysteine such RGD exposure elicits serum amyloid A3 expression and over-expression of matrix degrading enzymes and cytokines like MMP-13 (metalloproteinase-13), Ccl_5, Ccl_2, Cxcl10 and interleukin-6, substances otherwise known to hamper the proper collagen cross linking of bone matrix [10]. This group also reported that homocysteine increased the expression of genes for epigenetic DNA methylation like cytosine-5-methyl transferases1 (Dnmt1) and lymphoid specific helicase. The mechanism was found to be by increasing the expression of Fli1 (Friend leukemia virus integration 1), a transcription factor important for Dnmt1 stimulation. The authors also discovered that homocysteine caused hypermethylation of Lox (lysyl oxidase) proximal promoter that caused Lox repression. Lox is an extracellular copper dependent enzyme that catalyzes the formation of aldehydes from lysine residues in collagen precursors. In 2011, Lv et al. [11] reported a similar hypermethylation effect of homocysteine on promoter A region of estrogen receptor-alpha that cause repression of estrogen receptor alpha expression. The authors concluded that such inhibitory mechanisms can elicit postmenopausal osteoporosis in women, a bone disorder encountered by most females upon menopause. It was in the same year that Kriebitzsc et al. [12] established a link between homocysteine and vitamin D3. A microarray experiment by these authors on MC3T3-E1 murine pre-osteoblasts treated with 1,25-dihydroxyvitamin D_3 ($1,25(OH)_2D_3$) revealed the induction of a cluster of genes including the *cbs* (cystathionine β-synthase gene). Since CBS is an enzyme that converts homocysteine to cystathionine, thereby committing transsulfuration pathway to cysteine synthesis, the authors were intrigued to find out how vitamin D3 regulated the level of homocysteine in the osteoblast. They then discovered that *Cbs* mRNA levels were very much higher when osteoblasts obtained sufficient exposure to vitamin D3. Importantly, the chromatin immunoprecipitation on chip and transfection studies demonstrated a functional vitamin D response element in the second intron of *cbs*. The possible clinical relevance of these findings were investigated by these authors, and the human data from the Longitudinal Aging Study Amsterdam suggested a correlation between vitamin D status (25(OH)D$_3$ levels) and homocysteine levels. The authors drew conclusions that *cbs* is a primary 1,25(OH)$_2$D$_3$ target gene which renders homocysteine metabolism responsive to 1,25(OH)$_2$D$_3$.

In 2012, the role of homocysteine mediated endoplasmic reticulum (ER) stress in inducing apoptosis was reported revealing that osteoblast death can also occur during hyperhomocysteinemia. Homocysteine increases the expression of glucose-regulated protein 78, inositol-requiring transmembrane kinase and endonuclease 1α (IRE-1α), spliced X-box binding protein, activating transcription factor 4, and C/EBP homologous protein to carry out cell death [13].

Our group in 2013 reported how homocysteine altered the production of proteins in osteoblasts [14]. We were mainly interested in evaluating how homocysteine affected the synthesis of ligands like RANKL and OPG by osteoblasts. Proteins like RANKL, OPG and RANK (receptor on osteoclast) form a molecular trio which is one of the important regulators of bone remodeling. RANKL is required for RANK activation, development of multi-nucleated osteoclasts and induction of bone resorption. To regulate the osteoclast activity, the osteoblast also synthesizes OPG that serves as a decoy receptor for RANKL that binds it and prevents it from activating RANK. Our studies on how homocysteine affected the synthesis of OPG also threw light that this ligand production in osteoblast is coupled to the insulin-MAPK (mitogen activated protein kinase) signaling cascade and antioxidant defense machinery. The dephosphorylations of insulin receptor and associated downstream targets caused by homocysteine induce phosphorylation of PP2A (protein phosphatase 2A), a negative modulator of the insulin signaling. This increase in phosphatase activity also inhibited phosphorylation of p38 mitogen activated protein kinase, a pathway important for OPG synthesis by osteoblast cells. We were intrigued to find that dephosphorylations of insulin receptor signaling also produced increased nuclear translocation of ForkheadO1 transcription factor and activation of MnSod (manganese superoxide dismutase), an antioxidant. The RANKL synthesis however occurred independently and involved activation of c-Jun/JNK MAP kinase (JNK) signaling pathway. Thus the oxidative stress imparted by homocysteine altered the osteoblast behavior shifting the balance between bone formation and bone resorption.

1.2. Does homocysteine affect osteocytogenesis?

Osteocyte represents the third major cell type in the bone, which regulates the functions of osteoblasts and osteoclasts. These cells originate from mesenchymal stem cells via osteoblast lineage differentiation, and only 10–20% of such osteoblasts develop into osteocytes. Osteocytes also have an extraordinary long-life of 10–20 years and consequently constitute 95% of the cellular component of adult living bone. Mature osteocytes inhabit in cavities called "osteocyte lacunae" measuring some hundreds of μm^3 in volume that shape into an interconnected network *via* tiny canals or canaliculi to form the lacunar-canalicular pore system (LCS). LCS buried within the mineralized matrix positions osteocytes to derive nutrients from the blood supply, feel external mechanical signals, connect among themselves and with other cells on bone surfaces and control structural reorganization following bone remodeling [15, 16]. It was formerly thought that osteocytes are inert cells, however these are now contemplated to be superior cell type with endocrine functions. Upon stimulation, osteocytes secrete substances like RANK ligand, OPG, fibroblast growth factor23 (FGF23), prostanoids, nitric oxide, nucleotides, cytokines and growth factors that regulate bone remodeling. FGF23 produced by osteocytes regulate serum phosphate level by increasing renal phosphate excretion. Sclerostin and DKK1 specifically inhibit Wnt-B-catenin pathway that regulate bone formation [17, 18].

The process of "osteocytogenesis" is the evolution of a bone forming osteoblast to an osteocyte when it gets deeply buried in the bone matrix. The process involves three different phases: (*i*) type I osteoblastic-osteocyte, (*ii*) type II osteoid-osteocyte and (*iii*) type III preosteocyte (*surrounded by matrix*) [19]. Some of the noteworthy proteins involved in the process are: (a) Pdpn (E11), a trans-membrane glycoprotein that is required for the formation of dendrites, (b) osteocalcin, a non-collagenous protein for proper mineralization of marix, (c) dentine matrix protein or Dmp1 for regulation of crystal mineral size and osteocyte maturation [17, 20], (d) Phex, a metalloproteinase that binds to the inhibitor of Dmp1 *viz.* MEPE and regulates Dmp1 activity, (e) AHSG or FetuinA which regulates mineralization around developing osteocytes [21, 22] and (f) Sclerostin, a regulator of bone remodeling which can inhibit bone formation *via* downregulation of Wnt Lrp5/6 signaling, the major anabolic pathway in bone, which can activate osteoclasts and regulate mineralization [18, 23].

Till date there are only few reports that substantiate that osteocytes affected during hyperhomocysteinemia. One of the reasons for this is the difficulty in isolating osteocytes from mineralized tissues for obtaining these in sufficient numbers and purity. Over the years a cell line MLO-Y4 was developed by Lynda F Bonewald and many methods to isolate osteocytes from bone tissue were developed but none gave a complete picture as to how osteocytes responded to external stimuli. This is mainly because both the osteocytes and its extensive connections are not possible to be replicated in concert in vitro. Yet, investigations have been done on using the MLO-Y4 cell line to evaluate how osteocyte responds homocysteine. The results showed that homocysteine induced apoptosis in osteocyte culture via Nox and AMPK activation [24]. Nox or NADPH oxidase family of superoxide and hydrogen peroxide producing proteins represent an important source of reactive oxygen species whilst AMPK or adenosine monophosphate activated protein kinase is an energy sensor that regulates oxidative stress. The study by Takeno et al. did not render a complete picture as osteocytes are embedded deep inside the bone where it is not exposed to high concentrations of homocysteine. Thus we investigated how homocysteine affected osteocytes in vivo by administering mice with homocysteine i.p. and then evaluating how homocysteine in circulation modulated osteocytes employing microCT50, immunohistochemistry and Real Time PCR [25]. These techniques enabled us to identify time dependent changes in osteocyte lacunar numbers and osteocyte markers with onset of hyperhomocysteinemia. It was interesting to find that with induction of hyperhomocysteinemia, there was initially an increase in osteocyte lacunar numbers coupled to an increase in transcription and protein expression of many osteocyte markers.

But with time we observed that homocysteine mainly increased the protein expressions of Dmp1 and sclerostin that were otherwise involved in mineralization of osteocyte lacunae. This is in fact a pathogenic mechanism since increased mineralization is also a cause for bone instability. Another trait seen in these bone was osteocyte apoptosis. Erstwhile studies have previously demonstrated that apoptotic osteocytes are not "debris" but necessary regulators of a process called "targeted remodeling" wherein apoptotic osteocytes signal nearby cells to release factors like RANKL, VEGF, ATP, sphingosine-1-phosphate and chemokines for endothelial cell activation and recruitment of bone cell precursors, including osteoclasts and osteoblasts, to the site of injury to enable repair *via* BMU-mediated remodeling process [26, 27]. It has already been shown that homocysteine induces RANKL synthesis. Thus, homocysteine mediated induction of RANKL production by both osteoblasts and osteocytes is therefore an important determinant that drives bone to rapid bone resorption and thereby increased bone remodeling during hyperhomocysteinemia. Our findings thus provide an interesting avenue for future research into the role of osteocytes in disease-mediated changes in bone mineralization.

2. Conclusions

The effect homocysteine has on bone remodeling is dynamic. Unlike any other oxidant that generates free radicals, homocysteine exerts effects at multiple ways to induce cellular damage. We have seen that in some cases homocysteine induces gene methylations to render certain genes like Lox inactive so that collagen architecture is altered whereas in other cases homocysteine over expresses genes like Dmp and Sost to promote mineralization, a process that can produce adverse effects on long run. Understanding the complexities involved in hyperhomocysteinemia is therefore vital for designing therapeutics for treatment of bone disorders.

Author details

Viji Vijayan* and Sarika Gupta

*Address all correspondence to: vijivijayan7@gmail.com

Molecular Science Lab, National Institute of Immunology, New Delhi, India

References

[1] Robert K, Maurin N, Vayassettes C, Siauve N, Janel N. Cystathionine β-synthase deficiency affects mouse endochondral ossification. The Anatomical Record. Part A, Discoveries in Molecular, Cellular, and Evolutionary Biology. 2005;**282**:1-7. DOI: 10.1002/ar.a.20145

[2] Vacek TP, Kalani A, Voor MJ, Tyagi SC, Tyagi N. The role of homocysteine in bone remodeling. Clinical Chemistry and Laboratory Medicine. 2013;**51**:587-590. DOI: 10.1515/cclm-2012-0605

[3] Dayal S, Lentz SR. Murine models of hyperhomocysteinemia and their vascular phenotypes. Arteriosclerosis, Thrombosis, and Vascular Biology. 2008;**28**:1596-1605. DOI: 10.1161/ATVBAHA.108.166421

[4] Hermann M, Kraenzlin M, Pape G, Sand-Hill M, Herrman W. Relationship between homocysteine and biochemical bone turnover markers and bone mineral density in peri and post menopausal women. Clinical Chemistry and Laboratory Medicine. 2005;**43**:1118-1123. DOI: 10.1515/CCLM.2005.195

[5] Sakamoto W, Isomura H, Fujie K, Deyama Y, Kato A, Nishihira J, Izumi H. Homocysteine attenuates the expression of osteocalcin but enhances osteopontin in MC3T3E1 pre-osteoblastic cells. Biochimica et Biophysica Acta. 2005;**1740**:12-16. DOI: 10.1016/j.bbadis.2005.03.004

[6] Hermann M, Umanskaya N, Wildemann B, Colaianni G, Schmidt J, Widmann T, et al. Accumulation of homocysteine by decreasing the concentration of folate, vitamin B12, vitamin B6 does not influence the activity of human osteoblasts in vitro. Clinica Chimica Acta. 2007;**384**:129-134. DOI: 10.1016/j.cca.2007.06.016

[7] Hermann M, Umanskaya N, Widemann B, Colaianni G, Widmann T, Zallone A, Hermann W. Stimulation of osteoblast activity by homocysteine. Journal of Cellular and Molecular Medicine. 2008;**12**:1205-1210. DOI: 10.1111/j.1582-4934.2008.00104.x

[8] Thaler R, Spitzer S, Rumpler M, Fratzl-Zelman N, Klaushofer K, Paschalis EP, Varga F. Differential effects of homocysteine and beta-aminopropionitrile on pre-osteoblastic MC3T3E1 cells. Bone. 2010;**46**:703-709. DOI: 10.1016/j.bone.2009.10.038

[9] Thaler R, Agsten M, Spitzer S, Paschalis EP, Karlic H, Klushofer K, Verga F. Homocysteine suppresses the expression of collagen cross linker lysyl oxidase involving IL-6, Fli1 and epigenetic DNA methylation. Journal of Biological Chemistry. 2011;**286**:5578-5588. DOI: 10.1074/jbc.M110.166181

[10] Thaler R, Zwerina J, Rumpler M, Spitzer S, Gamsjaeger S, Paschalis EP, Klaushofer K, Varga F. Homocysteine induces serum amyloid A3 in osteoblasts via unlocking RGD-motifs in collagen. The FASEB Journal. 2013;**27**:446-463. DOI: 10.1096/fj.12-208058

[11] Lv H, Ma X, Che T, Chen Y. Methylation of promoter a of estrogen receptor alpha gene in hBMSC and osteoblasts and its correlation with homocysteine. Molecular and Cellular Biochemistry. 2011;**355**:35-45. DOI: 10.1007/s11010-011-0836-z

[12] Kriebitzsch C, Verlinden L, Eelen G, Van Schoor NM, Swart K, Lips P, et al. 1,25 dihydroxy vitamin D3 influences cellular homocysteine levels in murine pre-osteoblastic MC3T3E1 cells by direct regulation of cystathionine beta synthase. Journal of Bone and Mineral Research. 2011;**26**:2991-3000. DOI: 10.1002/jbmr.493

[13] Park S, Kim K, Kim W, Oh I, Cho C. Involvement of endoplasmic reticulam stress in homocysteine induced apoptosis of osteoblastic cells. Journal of Bone and Mineral Metabolism. 2012;**30**:474-484. DOI: 10.1007/s00774-011-0346-9

[14] Vijayan V, Khandelwal M, Manglani K, Singh RR, Gupta S, Surolia A. Homocysteine alters osteoprotegerin/RANKL system in the osteoblast to promote bone loss: Pivotal role of redox regulator forkhead O1. Free Radical Biology and Medicine. 2013;**61**:72-84. DOI: 10.1016/j.freeradbiomed.2013.03.004

[15] Dallas SL, Prideaux M, Bonewald LF. The osteocyte: An endocrine cell....And more. Endocrine Research. 2013;**34**:658-690. DOI: 10.1210/er.2012-1026

[16] Webster DJ, Schneider P, Dallas SL, Muller R. Studying osteocytes in their environment. Bone. 2013;**54**:285-295. DOI: doi.org/10.1016/j.bone.2013.01.004

[17] Beniash E, Deshpande AS, Fang P, Lieb W, Zhang X, Sfeir CS. Possible role of Dmp-1 in dentine mineralization. Journal of Structural Biology. 2011;**174**:100-106. DOI: 10.1016/j.jsb.2010.11.013

[18] Wijenayaka AR, Kogawa M, Lim HP, Bonewald LF, Findlay DM, Atkins GJ. Sclerostin stimulates osteocyte support of osteoclast activity by a RANKL dependent pathway. PLoS One. 2011;**6**:e25900. DOI: 10.1371/journal.pone.0025900

[19] Palumbo C, Palazzini S, Marotti G. Morphological study of intercellular junctions during osteocyte differentiation. Bone. 1990;**11**:401-406. DOI: 10.1016/8756-3282(90)90134-K

[20] Franz-Odendaal TA, Hall BK, Witten PE. Buried alive: How osteoblasts become osteocytes. Developmental Dynamics. 2006;**235**:176-190. DOI: 10.1002/dvdy.20603

[21] Seto J, Busse B, Gupta HS, Schafer C, Krauss S, Dunlop JWC, Masic A, Kerschitzki M, Zaslansky P, Boesecke P, et al. Accelerated growth plate mineralization and foreshortened proximal limb bones in Fetuin-a knockout mice. PLoS One. 2012;**10**:347333. DOI: 10.1371/journal.pone.0047338

[22] Rowe PSN. Regulation of bone-renal mineral and energy metabolism: The Phex, FGF-23, Dmp-1, MEPE ASARM pathway. Critical Reviews in Eukaryotic Gene Expression. 2013;**22**:61-86. DOI: 10.1615/ CritRevEukarGeneExpr.v22.i1.50

[23] van Bezooijen RL, ten Dijke P, Papapoulos SE, Lowik CW. SOST/sclerostin, an osteocyte derived negative regulator of bone formation. Cytokine & Growth Factor Reviews. 2005;**16**:319-327. DOI: 10.1016/j.cytogfr.2005.02.005

[24] Takeno A, Kanaazawa I, Tanae K, Notsu M, Yokomoto M, Yamaguchi T, Sugimoto T. Activation of AMP activated protein kinase protects against homocysteine induced apoptosis of osteocytic MLO-Y4 cells by regulating the expression of NADPH oxidase 1 (Nox1) and Nox2. Bone. 2015;**77**:135-141. DOI: 10.1016/j.bone.2015.04.025

[25] Vijayan V, Gupta S. Role of osteocytes in mediating bone mineralization during hyperhomocysteinemia. European Journal of Endocrinology. 2017;**233**:243-255. DOI: 10.1530/JOE-16-0562

[26] Weinstein RS, Nicholas RW, Manolagas SC. Apoptosis of osteocytes in glucocorticoid induced osteonectrosis of the hip. The Journal of Clinical Endocrinology and Metabolism. 2000;**85**:2907-2912. DOI: 10.1210/jcem.85.8.6714

[27] Cardoso L, Herman B, Verborgt O, Laudier D, Majeska RJ, Schaffler MB. Osteocyte apoptosis controls activation of intracortical resorption in response to bone fatigue. Journal of Bone and Mineral Research. 2009;**24**:597-605. DOI: 10.1359/jbmr.081210

www.ingramcontent.com/pod-product-compliance
Lightning Source LLC
Chambersburg PA
CBHW081244190326
41458CB00016B/5915